P9-CSC-683

the

ALL-NATURAL DIABETES COOKBOOK

THE WHOLE FOOD APPROACH TO GREAT TASTE AND HEALTHY EATING

JACKIE NEWGENT, RD

WEST HARRISON LIBRARY
2 Madison Street
West Harrison, NY 10604

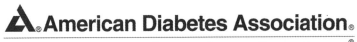

American Diabetes Association.

Cure • Care • Commitment®

Managing Editor, Book Publishing, Abe Ogden; *Acquisitions Editor, Consumer Books,* Robert Anthony; *Editor,* Laurie Guffey; *Production Manager,* Melissa Sprott; *Composition,* American Diabetes Association; *Cover Design,* Jody Billert; *Printer,* Transcontinental Printing.

©2007 by Jacqueline A. Newgent, RD. All Rights Reserved. No part of this publication may be reproduced or transmitted in any form or by any means, electronic or mechanical, including duplication, recording, or any information storage and retrieval system, without the prior written permission of the American Diabetes Association.

Printed in Canada
1 3 5 7 9 10 8 6 4 2

The suggestions and information contained in this publication are generally consistent with the Clinical Practice Recommendations and other policies of the American Diabetes Association, but they do not represent the policy or position of the Association or any of its boards or committees. Reasonable steps have been taken to ensure the accuracy of the information presented. However, the American Diabetes Association cannot ensure the safety or efficacy of any product or service described in this publication. Individuals are advised to consult a physician or other appropriate health care professional before undertaking any diet or exercise program or taking any medication referred to in this publication. Professionals must use and apply their own professional judgment, experience, and training and should not rely solely on the information contained in this publication before prescribing any diet, exercise, or medication. The American Diabetes Association—its officers, directors, employees, volunteers, and members—assumes no responsibility or liability for personal or other injury, loss, or damage that may result from the suggestions or information in this publication.

⊗ The paper in this publication meets the requirements of the ANSI Standard Z39.48-1992 (permanence of paper).

ADA titles may be purchased for business or promotional use or for special sales. To purchase more than 50 copies of this book at a discount, or for custom editions of this book with your logo, contact Lee Romano Sequeira, Special Sales & Promotions, at the address below, or at LRomano@diabetes.org or 703-299-2046.

For all other inquiries, please call 1-800-DIABETES.

American Diabetes Association
1701 North Beauregard Street
Alexandria, Virginia 22311

Library of Congress Cataloging-in-Publication Data
Newgent, Jackie.
  The all-natural diabetes cookbook : 150 high-flavor recipes made with real foods / Jackie Newgent.
    p. cm.
  Includes index.
  ISBN 978-1-58040-275-0 (alk. paper)
  1. Diabetes--Diet therapy--Recipes. 2. Cookery (Natural foods) I. Title.

RC662.N494 2007
641.5'6314--dc22

        2007011961

For my father, who has diabetes.

For my mother, who does most of his cooking.

CONTENTS

PREFACE

When I was a child, I loved to eat—and loved to eat often. I still do. My mother was a caterer and taught me about the importance of high-quality ingredients and the art of good cooking. Most of my earliest memories involve me, my mom, and food. Our house always had some marvelously savory aroma wafting about. Still, my favorite food was potato chips for quite a few years—high-quality ones, of course. Thankfully, I did enter adulthood with some healthful eating habits and amazing cooking and food lessons. I feel privileged to have learned so much about what "real food" is . . . and fortunate to realize how eating can and should be a pleasurable and important part of life. Today, my mother is still known by most in my hometown as being the best cook around. However, with no kids at home, just herself and my dad to cook for, and relaxing into her "wise" years, her cooking style at home has, frankly, become a bit less wise. Her food choices have become simpler and more convenient. And, though the finished recipes are still delicious, some ingredients that she's using aren't as "real" or "natural" as they once were. I wasn't overly worried about that until my father was diagnosed with diabetes.

Then, since my dad's health became a priority, I knew it was my job to help my mother whip up some new magic in the kitchen simply, conveniently, and naturally. I needed to create delicious recipes with ingredients my family loved. Finished dishes needed to be diabetes-friendly for my dad, while meeting my mother's high expectations for great taste and ease of preparation. And I wanted to share what I had learned about the importance of choosing natural and organically grown foods. The end result: *The All-Natural Diabetes Cookbook: The whole food approach to great taste and healthy eating.*

Making healthier food choices is an obstacle for some people with diabetes. One big reason: people don't want to give up flavor to eat better. But they shouldn't have to! *The All-Natural Diabetes Cookbook* provides everyday favorites for everyday people, with the addition of whole food nutrition and flavor, not subtraction of taste. More and more people are realizing they don't have to give up eating deliciously to eat nutritiously. They're learning how to choose natural, unprocessed foods. It's a trend that's growing, since using the freshest, least processed foods provides a way for people with diabetes (and their families) to eat healthfully, naturally, and deliciously—finally!

Today, natural cooking is a true passion of mine. So, whether you're just now learning diabetes-friendly cooking or have years of experience with it, I encourage you to take a taste tour with *The All-Natural Diabetes Cookbook*. I hope that natural cooking becomes a passion of yours—or at least an enjoyable part of your food life. I know you'll find these recipes enjoyable for everyone you know, with or without diabetes. I'm so pleased to have this opportunity to pass them on to my family—and to yours.

Jackie Newgent, RD

ACKNOWLEDGMENTS

I have many people to thank for their generous time, energy, and support of this project—and for helping me fully pursue my passion for great taste and healthy eating.

I'm grateful to:

My mother, for all she taught me about the importance of high-quality foods and the love of fine cooking.

My father, the true inspiration for this cookbook.

My bighearted sister, Rebecca Newgent, for her help in retesting several of the book's recipes, and my generous brother, Jim Newgent, for his creative, strategic thinking.

Amy Morse, for her gift of friendship, unique marketing mind, and help in making sure this cookbook gets into the hands of those who need it most.

My fabulous friends in New York for being so supportive—and understanding when I made my cookbook a priority. Tremendous thanks to Lisa Drayer, MA, RD; Lori Ferme; Leah McLaughlin; Patrick Kruchten; Alyssa Gelbard; Marnie Lobel; Jacinthe Babin;

Yanick Desmarais; Erika and Scott Pintoff; Rachel Sanzari, MS, RD; and Maye Musk, MS, RD.

The advice, recipe tips, and enthusiastic, long-distance encouragement sent from California, Ohio, Illinois, Maryland, Georgia, Arizona, Arkansas, Canada, Ireland, and Scotland, especially from Patricia Bannan, MS, RD; Sandi Newgent; Romy and Yves Bouhadana; Monica Barrock; Mary Ann Winner; Eric Oberman; Ken Chin; Michelle Novak; Scott and Maureen Heritage; Sang Min Lee; Ginette Desmarais; and John Graham.

My chef assistant, Lindsay deJongh, MS, RD, without whom I couldn't have completed this project.

Beth Shepard, my agent—and cheerleader.

My editors and the dedicated behind-the-scenes talent at the American Diabetes Association, including Rob Anthony, Abe Ogden, and Laurie Guffey.

Thanks so much to all!

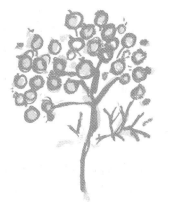

INTRODUCTION

The overriding food philosophy of *The All-Natural Diabetes Cookbook* is "fresh is best." I'll show you how to use natural ingredients, whole foods, and plenty of seasonal fresh fruits, vegetables, and herbs in your cooking, as well as fresh meats, seafood, and poultry. The primary focus of these recipes is on taste and nutrition. I also keep in mind that most people want recipes to be as fast and easy to make as possible. "Natural" convenience foods, like prepackaged salad greens or organic canned beans, help save time. Most recipes serve four and can be easily halved to serve two. Plus, nutritional facts accompany the recipes to help you fit them into your healthy meal plan.

ALL FOODS CAN FIT

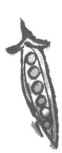

It's time to change the "good vs. bad" food philosophy a little. Overly processed, artificial, and saturated fat-laden foods are still not healthy. But you can include many more of your former favorites in a healthy meal plan than you once thought. Surprisingly, sugar, butter, and high-fat cheese are all used in this cookbook! When enjoyed in moderation, these foods can be part of a balanced, nutrient-rich meal plan for people with diabetes. And they can add so much enjoyment to healthful eating.

I'll show you how to include great-tasting ingredients in just the right quantities, using cooking techniques that maximize their flavor. Your job is to make sure you choose the most natural ingredients you can. An "all foods can fit" approach is at the heart of these recipes. It's the most realistic philosophy when it comes to healthy eating for a lifetime.

INGREDIENT HIGHLIGHTS

Since flavor is so important to me, I use ingredients differently than in the typical cookbook for people with diabetes. Here are some highlights.

- I use foods with "good" fats, such as extra virgin olive oil, avocados, and almonds, in the Mediterranean style. That means they're used more liberally than in typical low-fat diets. All my recipes have zero trans fat.
- I include butter and regular cheeses in small amounts when needed to make a dish rich and flavorful.
- I keep reduced-fat and other nutrient-modified foods to a minimum. I'll use them when they contain nothing artificial and when the dish's overall flavor appeal isn't affected by their use.
- I almost always use whole grains and other unrefined versions of foods. Occasionally I'll include naturally refined grains and refined grain products, such as ciabatta bread, for better taste, texture, or tradition. And I balance them with other ingredients to help them fit well into a healthy meal plan.
- I use honey and sugar in small amounts, since people with diabetes can enjoy sweets when they plan to include them.
- I call for plenty of fresh fruit and other nutritious, naturally sweet foods in these recipes.
- I don't use any artificial or nonnutritive sweeteners, keeping the recipes as natural as possible.
- I encourage the use of organic products. They're grown with fewer pesticides and chemicals, and are usually fresher and taste better. You can find organic versions of most foods and beverages these days.

BONUS FEATURES

You'll notice some bonus features throughout the recipes, too. There are easy-to-identify recipe symbols used throughout the cookbook to assure there's something to fit everyone's needs.

 is for quickest-to-fix dishes; they generally require 20 minutes or less to prepare—from start to finish.

 means the recipe is vegetarian—eggs and dairy may be included. Some recipes are suitable for vegans, too—no animal products included.

Each recipe may also have tips on choosing ingredients, cooking techniques, timesaving tricks, and party planning. These tips include:

- Fresh Fact
- Food Flair
- Fast Fix
- More Than Four?

WHAT'S NATURAL?

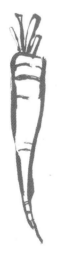 There's currently no standardized definition for the term "natural" that applies to all foods and beverages. The USDA has one for meat and poultry products: they can only be "natural" if they contain no artificial or synthetic ingredients and are minimally processed. While we wait for other products to be defined similarly, don't be misled by "natural" marketing gimmicks. My own goals in writing this book are that ingredients:

- Contain no artificial or synthetic ingredients, flavors, or colors, including no "bleached" ingredients
- Be no more than minimally processed
- Contain no hydrogenated fats and zero grams trans fat

- Contain no meat, poultry, eggs, or dairy products from animals given antibiotics*
- Contain no swordfish, shark, tilefish, king mackerel, or other fish with a high mercury content

*Choose products from animals raised without added growth hormones, if possible. However, by federal law, hormones aren't allowed to be given to poultry and hogs. So U.S. poultry (chicken and turkey) and pork are already free of added hormones.

WHAT'S ORGANIC?

Organic food is produced by farmers who emphasize the use of renewable resources and the conservation of soil and water to enhance environmental quality. It's produced without using most conventional pesticides; fertilizers made with synthetic ingredients or sewage sludge; bioengineering; or ionizing radiation. Organic meat, poultry, eggs, and dairy products come from animals that are given no growth hormones or antibiotics.

Look for the word "organic" and this seal to indicate organic packages of meat, cartons of milk or eggs, cheese, fresh produce, and other single-ingredient foods. Or you might see a sign above organic produce sections. For foods with more than one ingredient, you'll probably see percentages of organic ingredients included, such as "made with at least 70% organic ingredients."

The USDA Organic seal on food labels tells you that a product is either 100% organic or 95–100% organic. Though organic foods can be more costly than conventionally produced foods, I think you'll find them worth any added expense. You'll notice that I call for organic canned foods in this cookbook. That's a good place to start. Later, try adding organic frozen foods . . . organic produce can be next. Set a personal goal to make half of your food and beverage choices organic, if possible. Your body and taste buds will thank you.

NATURAL VS. ORGANIC

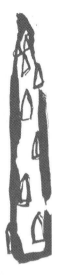

"Natural" and "organic" aren't the same thing. Organic refers to an agricultural growing method, not a health claim. Organic food differs from conventionally produced food in how it's grown, handled, and processed, but that doesn't mean it's always preservative-free or all-natural. Natural products are ideally free of added chemicals and preservatives, are minimally processed, and may have organic ingredients.

The idea is to aim to eat as naturally as possible. This will help assure that your body is getting the nutrients it needs, not the chemicals, calories, and fat it doesn't. Read all food labels carefully. When shopping for natural foods, don't automatically assume that you need to head to a health food store. The best-tasting products may come from small, local farmers who grow products and raise animals organically. Shop at nearby farmers' markets regularly. You'll have the highest quality ingredients at fair prices and wonderfully fresh, seasonal fruits, vegetables, herbs, meats, cheeses, and more.

Buy natural foods whenever you can. Buy organic foods selectively and whenever you can afford them. We'll all have more sustainable communities and more delicious, nutritious food on our plates. (For more information on buying natural foods, visit my website, *www.jackienewgent.com*.)

BEWARE OF THE DIRTY DOZEN

The USDA doesn't claim that organically produced food is more nutritious or safer than conventionally produced food. However, according to the Environmental Working Group (EWG), it's best to go organic when buying certain fruits and vegetables, as research finds it can reduce your exposure to chemicals found in conventionally produced food. The EWG has a list of the "dirty dozen," which is based on pesticide residues. So, try to choose organic when buying apples, bell peppers, celery, cherries, imported grapes, lettuce, nectarines, peaches, pears, potatoes, spinach, and strawberries.

ACHIEVING HIGH-FLAVOR DISHES NATURALLY

One of the missing components in many diabetes cookbooks is great flavor. Luckily, that's the highlight of *The All-Natural Diabetes Cookbook*. Below are 20 techniques that will help you love your food. Most of these tips are already incorporated into this cookbook, but use these suggestions at home to give your own recipes a high-flavor makeover.

1 **Be liberal with herbs.** Herbs are in the vegetable category, after all. For the freshest, fullest flavor, add fresh herbs toward the end of the cooking process or just before serving a dish.

2 **Spice it up.** Kick up flavors one spice at a time. Begin by adding 1/4 tsp of your spice of choice per recipe—and increase it from there.

3 **Marry in marinade.** Marinating ingredients to be cooked can help boost nutrition, tenderness, and taste. If you're marinating at room temperature, marinate for no more than two hours. Try marinating poultry in buttermilk or yogurt.

4 **Go nuts—and seeds.** Nuts and seeds add rich flavor, texture, visual appeal, and, well, nuttiness. Go for even more flavor by pan-toasting nuts and seeds first. Scatter roasted sunflower seeds or toasted almonds onto nearly any salad.

5 **Get saucy with it.** Even when recipes don't call for it, plop in a few drops of sauce, like soy sauce. It heightens flavor—and you might be able to cut out added salt. Sprinkle a few drops of Worcestershire, hot pepper, or naturally brewed soy sauce into low-sodium soups and stews.

6 **Drizzle and sizzle.** Experiment with aromatic oils, like toasted sesame, truffle, or hot chili oil. A little healthy fat can go a long way in added flair. Instead of butter or sour cream, drizzle truffle oil onto baked, roasted, or mashed potatoes.

7 **Say "cheese, please."** Top healthful dishes with high-flavored, high-fat ingredients, such as cheese. When it's so flavorful, very little is needed, making it easy to create a dish that's still healthful—and more enjoyable. Stir crumbled blue cheese or feta cheese into plain yogurt and use as a sandwich condiment.

8 **Use the yolk occasionally.** The yolk is the most nutrient-packed part of the egg—and the tastiest. Many mixed dishes will be a bit richer by adding an egg or by using one whole egg instead of two egg whites. Enrich lean ground chicken or turkey burger mixture with a whole beaten egg.

9 **Splash with acid.** Balance and uplift flavors with citrus juices, vinegars, or wines. Try matching by color. Lemon pairs well with fish; orange with chicken; red wine with beef. Add a few splashes of aged balsamic or red wine vinegar into bottled spaghetti sauce when simmering or to fresh tomato slices when serving.

10 **Reduce and seduce.** Reductions magnify flavor and can create thickness for a more seductive mouth feel. Simmer a creamy, low-sodium, low-fat carrot, butternut squash, or other veggie soup until it's extra thick. Use it as a sauce instead of a soup.

11 **Grill with flair.** Charcoal grilling is a popular cooking technique. It's healthful since no added fat is required. Make it more flavorful by adding woods, herbs, and spices to the coals. Grill boneless, skinless chicken breasts over aromatic woods, such as mesquite. Add rosemary twigs or cinnamon sticks, too.

12 **Brown it.** The browning of vegetables is called caramelization. Besides adding rich color, it adds a savory sweetness, too. Caramelize onions and serve on top of lean burgers, stir into steamed rice, or add to plain broth to make onion soup.

13 **Boost the beans.** Beans add good nutrition, fiber, and texture to meals. They're versatile, too. Plop canned beans into pasta sauce, soups, stews, salads, and stir-fry dishes. Use bean dips, like hummus, as a lovely sandwich spread. Mash cooked black beans and serve as a "bed" for entrées, like roast pork loin. (There's no need to rinse canned beans—which can remove a small amount of nutrients—unless you need to watch your sodium intake. In that case, rinse away—it can reduce the sodium content of the beans by 50%!)

14 **Be big with veggies.** Along with nutritional goodness, vegetables add texture, visual appeal, and natural savoriness (and sometimes sweetness) to meals. Enjoy veggies as entrées more often. Pile sandwiches high with raw or grilled veggies. Use low-sodium vegetable or tomato juice for preparation of whole wheat couscous, bulgur wheat, or brown rice.

15 **Flavor with fruit.** Fruits add texture, visual appeal, and natural sweetness—plus antioxidant nutrition. If a fruit is out of season, use frozen fruit since it's healthful, too. Serve salad topped with sliced pears or apples. Puree berries or other fruit with equal parts oil and vinegar to make a fruit vinaigrette. Make a salsa with diced peaches, onion, red bell pepper, and mint; serve with grilled fish or chicken.

16 **Make it hot, hot, hot.** A touch of "heat" takes flavor appeal to the next level. It adds more enjoyment to foods—especially those that are low in fat or sodium. Top grilled fish or lean poultry or meat with spicy salsas. Puree jalapeño pepper into hummus or other bean dips. Hot sauce can brighten the flavors of soups and most other savory foods.

17 **Whip it good.** Whipping up soft silken tofu in a blender creates a velvety smooth, soy-based flavor carrier and volume extender for sauces, salad dressings, dips, and more. While blending, add other flavorful ingredients, like balsamic vinegar and fresh basil, and use as a sandwich condiment, dip, or salad dressing.

18 **Eat tea.** Brew tea and use in vinaigrettes or as a poaching or other cooking liquid. It can add unique flavor and golden color. Use tea as the main ingredient in a marinade to help chicken breast develop a golden color.

UPPING UMAMI ♦ ♦ ♦ NATURALLY

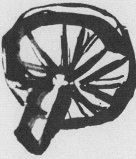

Umami is one of the five basic tastes (the others are sweet, salty, sour, and bitter). Umami is derived from the Japanese words umai, which means "delicious," and mi, which means "essence." Many people describe its taste as "meaty" or "savory." By including high-umami ingredients in healthful cooking, you'll naturally be adding savory satisfaction. Stock your kitchen with these foods rich in umami. Be sure to pick natural varieties of these foods, too.

- Aged balsamic vinegar
- Aged cheeses, including blue and Parmigiana-Reggiano cheese
- Beef
- Black beans
- Broth/stock, chicken and beef (reduced-sodium)
- Eggs
- Mushrooms, fresh and dried, such as morel, shiitake, and portabella
- Peas, fresh or frozen
- Red wine
- Sea vegetables (seaweeds)
- Seeds and nuts, including sunflower seeds and almonds
- Sauces, like Worcestershire, black bean, soy, and Asian fish sauces
- Shellfish and dark-fleshed fish, including salmon and anchovies
- Soy products, including miso and tofu
- Tomatoes and tomato products
- Truffle oil

 19 **Up the umami.** Umami is considered the fifth taste. It adds scrumptious savoriness to foods. Be sure to stock your kitchen with naturally rich, high-umami foods—and be sure to use them (see sidebar).

20 **Allow overnight mingling.** Cooking in advance and refrigerating overnight allows flavors to mingle in many mixed dishes. And it saves time on the day you plan to serve the food. Leftovers can be lovable, too. Make creamy chicken salads or chilled, grain-based salads the day before you plan to eat them.

33 NATURAL, NO-FUSS COOKING AND BAKING TIPS

Some people are worried that cooking more healthfully will take more time. It doesn't have to! Most recipes in *The All-Natural Diabetes Cookbook* are already quick to fix. And here are 33 suggestions you can use at home to make your own recipes speedier or easier to prepare.

1 **Gather your mis en place** [MEEZ ahn plahs]. This is a French cooking term that means "everything in its place." Measuring or portioning ingredients in advance, and organizing them in the order that you need them, will make your efforts more efficient and enjoyable. It works for me!

2 **Pick nonstick.** Using nonstick cookware can help prevent foods from sticking, making cooking and clean-up less stressful. Natural cooking spray can help, too. Make your own cooking spray if you can—you'll need to buy a pump-spray bottle and select the oil. And for best results, consider spraying the food, not the pan, when you can.

3 **Skinny-size it.** The skinnier the ingredients to be cooked, the speedier the cooking process. For instance, make paillards by pounding pieces of poultry, meat, or firm fish until very thin for quicker sautéing or grilling-—and more plate coverage. Choose skinny, pencil-like asparagus stalks instead of those as thick as your thumb.

4 **Mix it up.** Create pancake, cookie, muffin, or spice mixes when you have a spare moment, so you'll save time when ready to fix. Create several batches at once, too. Make your own pancake mix by measuring flours, baking powder, and salt; make oatmeal cookie mix by measuring oats, flour, baking powder, and salt. Label, date, and store each mix in a well-sealed plastic bag or jar for weeks.

5 **Freeze for ease.** When fruits, like raspberries, aren't in season, or you don't want to mess with peeling or slicing whole fruit, use frozen fruits. They're a nutritious substitute for fresh fruit. The same applies to veggies like peas or corn, also.

6 **Love your leftovers.** Even when recipes call for freshly prepared ingredients, leftovers will often work perfectly—and be speedier. Chicken salad, for instance, tastes wonderful using roasted chicken leftovers. If it's already seasoned, just adjust other seasonings in the recipe accordingly. Also, a grilled veggie sandwich is delicious made with vegetables grilled two minutes, two hours, or two days in advance.

7 **Don't kick the can.** Use organic canned beans, tomatoes, or corn to save time. These foods are canned when in-season, at their peak of ripeness, nutritional value, and flavor. When going organic, there's usually just water and sometimes salt or sea salt added. So, it's still natural. And it can be more nutritious than fresh produce that's out of season—or had to travel hundreds of miles to reach you.

8 **Befriend your butcher.** Befriend your fish monger, too. He or she can cut roasts and steaks "to order" for you. All of the guesswork and trimming time is taken care of for you. It'll cut the need for an extra cutting board at prep time, as well.

9 **Similar-size it.** When ingredients are about the same size, they can be cooked about the same length of time. That's true from cookies to kebabs and poultry to potatoes. One example: if you're roasting baby potatoes, but some aren't baby-sized, cut them into similar-size pieces or halve the largest ones. This'll provide more even—and faster—cooking.

10 **Do it yourself.** Don't spend too much time hunting at the supermarket for specialty ingredients. Make your own versions. For instance, add a few drops of hot pepper sauce to regular Dijon mustard to create spicy mustard. Stir a little honey into regular mustard to create honey mustard.

11 **Use utensils wisely.** Use a chef's knife instead of dirtying a food processor for small chopping tasks. Choose a small ice cream or cookie scoop for forming perfectly sized meatballs. Try a grapefruit spoon for super-easy tomato or melon scooping.

12 **Don't do it yourself.** A growing number of prepackaged, prewashed, presliced, and preportioned food choices are now available. They're ideal when time is of the essence. But be sure to buy those that are natural, too. Prepackaged baby spinach, pregrilled chicken breast pieces, and single-serve milk cartons and yogurt containers are all popular time-saving picks.

13 **Give into commercials.** Some major food companies have natural foods. So, don't judge a food just by company name. Foods that are TV commercial stars may be healthful, too. They can help expand the array of choices available to you—and save specialty shopping time.

14 **Fill the fridge.** Many ingredients, parts of recipes, and entire recipes can be made one, two, or three days in advance. Bake potatoes, wrap, and chill. They're ready for reheating or using in a mashed potato recipe any time for the next couple of days. Slice or dice veggies, like bell peppers, onions, and zucchini, up to a day before you need them. Keep well sealed and chilled. Prepare and refrigerate soups, sauces, and stews uncovered, overnight. Fat solidifies on top when chilled—which you can then remove.

15 **Mix 'n' mingle.** Some foods are actually tastiest when cooked ahead of time and refrigerated overnight. It allows for flavors to mingle— and frees up your time the day you plan to serve the food. Sauces, spreads, and dips are good examples. It's true of pasta, tuna, and chicken salad, too. Be sure to add any crunchy items, like nuts, just before serving.

16 **Chill out.** Baked goods are generally good candidates for freezing. And when you package them individually, it'll be easier to eat just one serving instead of being tempted by more. So, bake and freeze muffins, cookies, cupcakes, brownie squares, and cake slices. Place one packaged serving on the counter at room temperature in the morning and it'll be ready to enjoy in the evening.

17 **Cheat!** Go ahead and take it easy on yourself when cooking—cheating's not always a bad idea! Grab a rotisserie chicken from the grocery store, remove the skin, and pull the chicken from the bone to use in a quick-cooking recipe.

18 **Let it lie.** Having a lazy, stay-at-home Sunday? If so, take a few minutes and prepare items that can be stored in airtight containers and kept on the counter for the week. Pan-toast nuts. Bake homemade granola. Premix dry ingredients for pancakes, muffins, and more.

19 **Marinate in minutes.** Often a marinade is mostly for flavoring, not tenderizing. When that's the case, use half of it to marinate in minutes, rather than hours. Use the other half as a basting liquid during cooking or dipping sauce at the table. (Just make sure you never re-use marinade the meat's been soaking in.)

 Procrastinate. When a recipe seems lengthy, do some of it today and save some of it for tomorrow. Review the recipe first to determine what can be done in advance.

 Grill in. Too cold outside, no gas in the tank, or no desire to mess with charcoal briquettes? Grill inside, not out. There are indoor electric and gas grills, grill pans, and panini-style grills from which to choose. Whichever you use depends on what you plan to grill. Broiling is a speedy alternative, too.

22 **Have a two-way.** Grain dishes are often tasty served hot or cold. Couscous, quinoa, and bulgur side dishes are prime examples. Serve it hot the first day, then chill the leftovers. The next day, squirt the dish with fresh lemon juice and serve it as a cool side salad.

23 **Be boring.** Variety isn't always the spice of life. When a recipe calls for four types of beans, three types of bell peppers, or two types of berries, it's often for color variety. But these recipes will still taste good with one type of bean, bell pepper, or berry. It'll save shopping time, prep time, and maybe money, too.

Spend money, save minutes. If you put a dollar value on your time, it can be cheaper in the long run to purchase certain specialty products. For instance, instead of making homemade yogurt cheese, spend the extra few dimes on store-bought Greek yogurt—no straining required.

 Thaw while you sleep. When a recipe calls for a frozen item to be thawed, don't wait until you're preparing the recipe to do so. Zapping it in the microwave can create a partially thawed, partially cooked, partially still-frozen mess. And thawing on the counter is unsafe for many foods. Instead, thaw items overnight in the fridge while you're dreaming. It'll help prevent a potential nightmare at prep time.

 Do two (or three) things at once. Make good use of your time when cooking. Review recipes in advance to determine what should be done first, what can wait for last, and what can be done at the same time. Often while something is cooking, other parts of a recipe or meal can be gathered, measured, and prepped.

 Take a shortcut. Why buy two ingredients when you can buy one? When a recipe calls for salsa and jalapeño chili pepper, skip the jalapeño and use a spicy salsa instead. If a recipe suggests a mixture of white and dark meat, just use white—and save some calories, too.

 Make more. If you're a fan of a certain food, make extra one day to have available for recipes for the next day or two. If you're a pasta fan, for instance, cook double the noodles. Serve half of it at dinner; toss the other half with a little olive or canola oil, loosely cover, and chill. Use for a pasta salad for lunch or another pasta dish for dinner the next day.

Eat outside the box. Don't always think of eggs or oatmeal as breakfast food, or pasta or steak as dinner food. Mix things up. Eggs are easy to fix—and can be part of an absolutely delicious dinner. Leftover pasta can be a balanced breakfast for those willing to think outside the traditional meal box.

30 **Go off-recipe.** For baked dessert recipes, you need to be pretty precise with measurements. But most other recipes don't usually need to be followed to a tee. For instance, if you can't find heirloom tomatoes, go with vine-ripened beefsteak tomatoes. If you don't like olives, replace them with sun-dried tomatoes. If you need to limit salt, don't add all of the salt called for in a recipe—up the herbs instead. Make each recipe your own. And have fun in the process, too.

31 **Think outside the recipe.** A soup can also be a gravy. An appetizer can be a salad. And so on. A creamy chestnut soup is a delicious soup, but it's a unique gravy for turkey or mashed potatoes. Serve some beef or chicken satays as appetizers, then cube some of the satay meat and serve in a salad. When one recipe works as two, it saves time—and can add intrigue to meals.

32 **Make it a family affair.** Have the entire family pitch in to prepare meals. Kids are more apt to eat healthful foods when they have a role in preparation, too. It's a fun activity. And it'll provide more time to be together as a family—during meal preparation and at mealtime.

33 **Outsource your cooking.** If you have cash to spare, hire a personal chef. Request recipes you'd like her to make from *The All-Natural Diabetes Cookbook*, too. That's called fuss-free cooking, for sure!

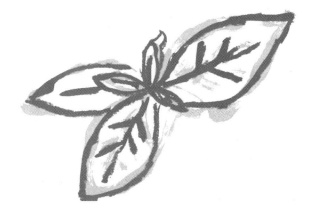

THE ALL-NATURAL, DIABETES-FRIENDLY SUBSTITUTION LIST

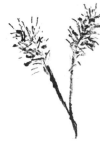

To make a recipe healthier, ingredient substitutions for cooking or baking are not necessarily tasty substitutions. For instance, using fat-free mayonnaise instead of regular mayonnaise will decrease fat, but will also decrease flavor satisfaction. And, unfortunately, these changes can add preservatives or other not-so-real ingredients that your body doesn't need.

Below is a sampling of 10 simple, yet succulent swaps to try at home—naturally. Most of these swaps (and many more) are already used within the recipes of *The All-Natural Diabetes Cookbook*.

INSTEAD OF	TRY
1/4 cup sour cream	1/4 cup low-fat or fat-free plain Greek yogurt (or yogurt cheese; see recipe, page 63)
2 Tbsp mayonnaise (for salads)	1 Tbsp mayonnaise + 1 Tbsp plain, low-fat or fat-free Greek or regular yogurt + pinch of lemon zest or splash of hot pepper sauce
2 Tbsp mayonnaise (on sandwiches)	1 Tbsp guacamole or mashed avocado or 2 Tbsp hummus or bean dip
1 Tbsp butter (in baking or sautéing)	1 1/2 tsp canola, olive, or other heart-friendly oil + 1 tsp butter
1 cup sugar (in baking)	3/4 cup turbinado sugar + pinch of sweet spice, such as ground cinnamon, and/or extra 1/4 tsp vanilla extract

INSTEAD OF	TRY
1 oz regular cheese	3/4 oz high-flavored regular cheese, such as extra sharp cheddar instead of mild cheddar cheese
1 oz chocolate	3 Tbsp unsweetened natural cocoa powder + 1 Tbsp canola oil
1 cup bleached all-purpose flour (in baking)	1/2 cup unbleached all-purpose flour + 1/3 cup whole wheat flour
1 tsp salt	1/2 tsp sea salt + up to twice the amount of herbs or spices already in recipe
1/4 cup vinaigrette	1/4 cup natural low-fat vinaigrette or puree of 1/4 cup cubed fruit + 1 Tbsp oil + 1 Tbsp vinegar

WHAT'S IN SEASON?

When produce is in season, it's at its peak of ripeness, nutritional value, and flavor. (It's usually least expensive then, too!) While you can find most produce all year long, different varieties of fruits and vegetables peak at different times of the year . . . seasonality and availability will vary in different parts of the country, too.

Keep in mind, if you're having difficulty finding a certain fresh fruit or vegetable, it may be out of season in your area. When out of season locally, it's often better to purchase frozen, not fresh. Frozen produce is picked and frozen at its peak of ripeness, nutritional value, and flavor. See page 303 to find the best time to purchase many popular picks fresh—and at their seasonal best.

FRESH HERB MATCHES

Fresh herbs can add lovely flavor, nutrition, and overall appeal to a dish, but only if you match them well with foods. By using the freshest herbs, you'll be able to use less fat or sodium in a dish. Try some of my all-time favorite herb pairings below.

Basil Beans, bread (savory), cheese, eggs, fish, fruits, lamb, pasta, poultry, rice
Vegetables: asparagus, broccoli, cauliflower, celery, cucumbers, eggplant, green beans, onions, parsnips, peas, potatoes, salad greens, spinach, tomatoes

Cilantro Avocado, chili
Vegetables: corn, salad greens, tomatoes

Chives Beef, cheese, eggs, fish, ham, poultry, rice, soups/stews
Vegetables: asparagus, beets, Brussels sprouts, carrots, corn, cucumbers, potatoes, salad greens, summer squash, tomatoes

Dill Bread (savory), fish, poultry, seafood
Vegetables: asparagus, beets, broccoli, carrots, cabbage, corn, cucumbers, green beans, peas, potatoes, tomatoes, summer squash

Mint Chocolate, lamb, pork
Vegetables: corn, cucumbers, green beans, peas, potatoes, tomatoes

Oregano Beans, beef, bread (savory), fish, lamb, pasta, rabbit, soups/stews
Vegetables: asparagus, broccoli, corn, eggplant, green beans, mushrooms, onions, peas, potatoes, summer squash, tomatoes

Parsley Beans, cheese, eggs, fish, lamb, pasta, pork (including ham), poultry, rice, seafood, soups/stews
Vegetables: artichokes, beets, cabbage, carrots, celery, corn, cucumbers, mushrooms, onions, parsnips, peas, potatoes, salad greens, summer squash, tomatoes, turnips

Rosemary Beans, bread (savory), poultry, fish, lamb, pasta
Vegetables: broccoli, corn, green beans, parsnips, peas, potatoes, turnips, summer squash

Sage Cheese, lamb, poultry, rice, soup/stews, venison
Vegetables: Brussels sprouts, corn, eggplant, sweet potatoes, tomatoes, winter squash

| Tarragon | Cheese, eggs, fish, lamb, pasta, pears, pork (including ham), poultry, rice, seafood, soups/stews |

Tarragon — Cheese, eggs, fish, lamb, pasta, pears, pork (including ham), poultry, rice, seafood, soups/stews
Vegetables: asparagus, carrots, cauliflower, celery, corn, dark leafy greens, eggplant, green beans, mushrooms, peas, potatoes, salad greens, summer squash, tomatoes, winter squash

Thyme — Beans, beef, eggs, fish, pork, poultry, soups/stews
Vegetables: asparagus, carrots, cauliflower, celery, corn, cucumbers, dark leafy greens, eggplant, onions, summer squash, sweet potatoes, tomatoes, winter squash

SPICE IS NICE

While it's always fun to experiment with spices in cuisine, too much spice can kill a dish—and your taste buds. So try one spice, about 1/4 tsp at a time. Next time, go for more of the same spice—or try using two. Here are some of my favorite spices, along with the foods they go with best.

Allspice — Bread (sweet), fruits (especially apple, cherries), meats, poultry
Vegetables: cabbage, carrots, parsnips, peas, sweet potatoes, tomatoes, turnips, winter squash

Cardamom — Bread (sweet), fruits (especially apple, cherries), ham
Vegetables: cabbage, mushrooms, sweet potatoes, winter squash

Chili powder — Avocado, chili, eggs, rice
Vegetables: corn, cauliflower, green beans, tomatoes

Cinnamon — Bread (sweet), chili, fruit (especially apple, cherries), meats, oats, rice
Vegetables: beets, carrots, corn, sweet potatoes, winter squash

Cumin — Beans, beef, cheese, eggs, fish, ham, pasta, poultry, rice, seafood, soups/stews
Vegetables: cabbage, corn, cucumbers, eggplant, green beans, sweet potatoes, tomatoes, winter squash

Curry powder — Eggs, poultry, ham, pasta, rice, seafood
Vegetables: broccoli, cabbage, carrots, cauliflower, parsnips, peas

Fennel seed — Bread (savory/sweet), cheese, eggs, fish, onions, pasta, pork, rice
Vegetables: cabbage, celery, onions, peas, potatoes

Ginger Bread (sweet), fish, fruits (especially apple, orange, peach), pork (including ham), poultry, rice
Vegetables: asparagus, beets, cabbage, carrots, sweet potatoes, tomatoes, winter squash

Mace Beef, bread (savory/sweet), cheese, fruits (especially apple, cherries), pork (including ham), poultry
Vegetables: beets, broccoli, Brussels sprouts, cabbage, cauliflower, carrots, celery, corn, dark leafy greens, eggplant, parsnips, sweet potatoes, turnips, winter squash

Nutmeg Bread (sweet), cheese, fruits (especially apple, cherries), pork, poultry
Vegetables: asparagus, broccoli, cabbage, cauliflower, dark leafy greens, eggplant, green beans, mushrooms, onions, parsnips, potatoes, sweet potatoes, tomatoes, winter squash

Saffron Beans, bread (savory/sweet), fish, pasta, poultry, rice, seafood, soups/stews
Vegetables: corn, cucumbers

MARVELOUS MENUS: 16 SIMPLE, SEASONAL, AND SCRUMPTIOUS MEALS

Pick your season . . . then pick a menu. Many are ideal for special occasions. But don't feel you need to stick to the meal theme. Sit down to a holiday dinner any day. Celebrate Fat Tuesday on a Wednesday. Have a Super Bowl feast while watching the Academy Awards. Each deliciously easy menu includes one serving of a fabulous recipe from this cookbook.

SPRING Lovely Ladies Luncheon
This is ideal to serve for Mother's Day—but men will enjoy this beautifully balanced meal, too.

- **Caramelized Anjou Pear, Sage, and Gorgonzola Quesadilla** (see page 82)
- 3 oz roasted chicken breast
- 1 cup each steamed broccoli and cauliflower florets

Spring Break Breakfast

Take a vacation from your breakfast routine with this sunny start to your day—even if it's a not-so-sunny day.

- **Blanco Huevos Rancheros** (see page 36)
- 1 fresh peach
- 1/4 cup organic low-fat cottage cheese

Cinco de Mayo Fiesta

Celebrate this spring holiday with a little sangria, too.

- 2 cups baby spinach salad with 1–2 Tbsp natural low-fat raspberry or other fruity vinaigrette
- **Tequila–Lime Chicken with Spinach Fettucine in Creamy Jalapeño Sauce** (see page 216)
- 1 cup cooked sliced red or yellow bell peppers

Memorial Day Dinner

Add worldly flair to your next meal with a bountiful bowl of interesting flavors, colors, and textures. Don't forget the chopsticks. And, if you can, sip a spirit with your soba.

- 2 cups baby arugula or field green salad with 1–2 Tbsp natural low-fat balsamic vinaigrette
- **Asian Sesame Soba Noodle Bowl with Bell Peppers and Snow Peas** (see page 212)
- 2 oz grilled lean filet mignon, thinly sliced and served on top of the noodles

SUMMER Beach Bag Lunch

Headed to the beach? You'll be refreshed by this light Mediterranean lunch. No utensils are required.

- **Stuffed Lemony Hummus Pita** (see page 208)
- 1 cup English (hothouse) cucumber slices with skin
- 1/2 cup cherry or grape tomatoes
- 10 unsalted almonds or 1/2 oz nut mixture
- 1 fresh plum or fig

Red, White, & Blue Cookout
Celebrate your Independence Day with fireworks for your palate.
- 1-oz slice low-fat blueberry bread or muffin
- 3 oz spice-rubbed grilled wild salmon
- 10 grilled cherry tomatoes on skewers
- 10 grilled white onion wedges on skewers, brushed with 1 tsp extra virgin olive oil
- **Balsamic Strawberries** (see page 288)

It's Too Hot to Cook
Who needs soup and salad—or sandwich and salad? How about salad and salad? Better yet, try this salad, salad and salad!
- **Bow Tie Macaroni Salad** (see page 152)
- 2 cups baby field green salad with 1–2 Tbsp natural low-fat balsamic or raspberry vinaigrette
- 1 cup mixed berries fruit salad

Right-Sized Bikini and Swim Trunk Meal
Need to squeeze into that bathing suit? Just dive into these light, yet luscious bites and you won't need to fret about its itsy-bitsy-ness.
- 1/2 cup shelled edamame
- **Fresh Tarragon Chicken Salad with Almonds on Marble Rye** (see page 186)
- 15 red seedless grapes

AUTUMN ### Fall Fruit Harvest Breakfast
Savor a fresh fall fruit in each bite. Kids will even give this brightly flavored meal an "A" as their back-to-school breakfast favorite.
- **Granny Smith Breakfast Sausage Patties** (see page 48)
- 1 piece whole wheat toast with 1 Tbsp mashed banana
- 1/2 cup plain, fat-free yogurt stirred with 3 Tbsp mashed banana and 1/2 cup blueberries

Spooky Halloween Supper

Here's a scary, yet lip-smacking dinner for this trick-filled holiday.

- **Simple Gazpacho** (call it "Chilled Blood Sipper"; see page 178)
- 1 boiled egg, halved, lightly drizzled with 2 tsp organic ketchup (call it "Screaming Eyeballs")
- 1 cup organic low-fat vegetarian chili, served with a cinnamon stick (call it "Witch's Goulash")
- 5 large black olives (for your fingertips!)

Election Night Nibbles

Go vote! Then plan on a no-cook dinner that's ideal for grazing, tapas-style, throughout the exciting (or frustrating) election night news coverage.

- 6 cooked, chilled, large shrimp with 2 Tbsp cocktail sauce
- 1/2 oz soy chips or crisps, flavor of choice, or plantain chips
- 1 cup raw veggie sticks, such as jicama and mixed bell peppers
- 1 small apple or pear
- 1 oz unsalted nut mixture
- **Pomegranate Martini** (to toast the winners—or losers! see page 281)

Thanksgiving Dinner Anytime

Thanksgiving is such a delicious day. Enjoy its flavors any time you wish, with family or friends you're thankful to have.

- **Creamy Chestnut Soup** (see page 166)
- 3 oz roasted, sliced turkey breast with 2 tsp cranberry sauce
- 1/2 cup mashed pumpkin or sweet potato with 1/2 tsp butter
- 1 cup steamed green beans with 1 Tbsp unsalted, sliced, pan-toasted almonds

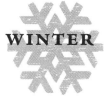

WINTER Hometown Holiday Dinner

Lean meat or poultry doesn't need to be doused in gravy. It's mouth-watering when served on this memorable bean "bed." Best of all, this holiday meal includes a perfectly portioned slice of pie.

- 3 oz roasted or broiled lean lamb chop or poultry breast, seasoned to taste
- **Stewed Rosemary Bean Bed** (see page 248)
- 1 cup roasted, sliced beets, splashed with 1 tsp aged balsamic vinegar
- 1 thin slice pumpkin pie

Savory Super Bowl Party Feast

You can root for all the players on this party buffet. It's a touchdown for your taste buds.

- **Minted Middle Eastern Meatballs** (see page 100)
- 1/2 whole wheat pita
- 1 cup raw broccoli florets or other veggies with 1–2 Tbsp natural Ranch salad dressing
- 1/2 oz blue corn tortilla chips with 2 Tbsp salsa

Not-So-Fat Tuesday Plate

You'll get jazzed up about this New Orleans-inspired meal.

- 2 1/2 oz lean baked natural ham, oven-heated or pan-grilled, sprinkled with 2 tsp chopped pecans and 1 tsp maple syrup
- 1 cup steamed kale, Swiss chard, or spinach with a lemon wedge, seasoned to taste
- **Creole Fingerling Potato Salad** (see page 122)

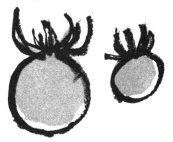

Valentine's Dinner for Couples (or Singles)

Ladies, this will be a pleasing meal for your partner . . . guys, same goes for you!

- 2 cups baby spinach salad with 1/2 cup artichoke hearts, 1–2 Tbsp natural low-fat balsamic or red wine vinaigrette, and 1/2 Tbsp pan-toasted pine nuts
- **Eye of Round Steak with Organic Red Wine Reduction Sauce** (see page 222)
- 1 cup steamed wild mushrooms sprinkled with 1/2 tsp extra virgin olive oil and fresh thyme leaves
- 6 steamed baby carrots
- 1/2 cup cooked bulgur or whole wheat couscous with 1/2 Tbsp pan-toasted pine nuts

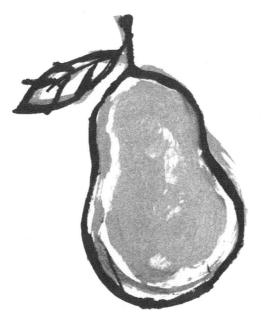

THE
NATURAL
RECIPE
COLLECTION

RISE 'N' SHINE

BLUE RIBBON BLUEBERRY MUFFINS

Serves 12/serving size: 1 muffin

No need to hunt for a blue ribbon-winning muffin recipe that'll easily fit into your healthful eating plan. This is it. These blueberry-loaded muffins are just the right size, too.

- 1 cup vanilla soy milk
- 2 Tbsp unsalted butter, melted
- 1 large egg
- 1/2 tsp fresh lemon zest (grated peel)

- 1/2 tsp pure almond extract
- 3/4 cup turbinado sugar
- 1 2/3 cups unbleached all-purpose flour

- 1 1/2 tsp double-acting baking powder
- 3/4 tsp sea salt
- 2 (1/2-pint) containers fresh blueberries (about 2 cups)

DIRECTIONS

1. Preheat the oven to 375°F. Spray 12 cups of a nonstick muffin tin with natural butter-flavored cooking spray, or place 12 muffin liners into the cups of a muffin tin.

! FRESH FACT

Local blueberries are in season in spring and summer. These muffins will taste best then, too. However, if you bake these in the fall or winter, use frozen, organic, thawed blueberries in the batter. The frozen berries are still loaded with antioxidants. Of course, the most important thing to do when it comes to blueberries is to eat them—any which way you can.

2. In a large bowl, vigorously whisk the soy milk with the butter until combined. Whisk in the egg, lemon zest, and almond extract until combined, then whisk in the sugar. In a medium bowl, sift together the flour, baking powder, and salt. Stir the flour mixture into soy milk mixture until just combined. Fold in the blueberries.

3. Divide batter among 12 muffin cups, about 1/3 cup batter per muffin cup. Bake 20 minutes or until firm and springy to the touch. Cool in the pan on a rack. After at least 20 minutes, run a small, flexible spatula or butter knife around the muffin edges and gently remove. Serve at room temperature, chilled, or semi-frozen.

Exchanges: 2 carbohydrate; 150 calories, 24 calories from fat, 3 g total fat, 1 g saturated fat, 25 mg cholesterol, 230 mg sodium, 28 g total carbohydrate, 1 g dietary fiber, 15 g sugars, 3 g protein.

FAST FIX

Bake and freeze these marvelous morsels. Just place a muffin into a covered container at room temperature overnight and it'll be ready to eat in the morning. Or just take a muffin out of the freezer in the morning and enjoy it semi-frozen or chilled. When you eat the muffin semi-frozen, the blueberries inside taste like little mini blueberry popsicles.

FOOD FLAIR

To up the fiber and add an earthier flair to this morning muffin, use 1 cup unbleached all-purpose flour and 2/3 cup buckwheat flour. This will boost your whole grain intake, too.

Fold in all but 12 of the blueberries. After dividing batter among the muffin cups, press a blueberry on top of each.

BUCKWHEAT BANANA PANCAKES WITH WALNUTS

Serves 4/serving size: 2 pancakes

These hearty pancakes contain buckwheat flour. You might be surprised to know that buckwheat is not wheat at all; it's an herb of Russian descent. So, perhaps a better name for these pancakes may be Russian roulettes.

- 1/4 cup buckwheat flour
- 3 Tbsp unbleached all-purpose flour
- 1 tsp double-acting baking powder
- 1/2 tsp sea salt
- 2 tsp cold, unsalted butter, cut into pieces
- 1 tsp acacia or other mild floral honey
- 1 large egg
- 1/2 cup vanilla soy milk
- 2 large fully ripened bananas, peeled
- 2 Tbsp chopped walnuts

DIRECTIONS

1. In a medium bowl, combine the flours, baking powder, salt, butter, and honey into a finely crumbled mixture with a pastry blender or potato masher.

2. In a large bowl, whisk together the egg and soy milk. Add the flour mixture to the soy milk mixture and whisk until well combined. Let stand for 5 minutes. Mash one banana and set aside; very thinly slice the other banana and stir the slices into the batter.

3. Lightly coat a large flat skillet or griddle with natural cooking spray (see Fresh Fact) and place over medium heat. Spoon about 1/4 cup batter per pancake on the hot skillet. Cook pancakes in batches for 2 minutes per side or until lightly browned. Keep cooked pancakes warm on a plate loosely covered with foil. Serve pancakes topped with mashed bananas and walnuts.

Exchanges: 1 starch, 1 fruit, 1 fat; 180 calories, 58 calories from fat, 6 g total fat, 2 g saturated fat, 60 mg cholesterol, 450 mg sodium, 27 g total carbohydrate, 3 g dietary fiber, 11 g sugars, 5 g protein.

FRESH FACT

You can make your own natural cooking spray with your favorite oil—olive, canola, soybean, peanut, or more. Just purchase a pump-spray bottle, fill, and spray—naturally!

FAST FIX

Create your own pancake mix. Stir together the flours, baking powder, and salt, and store in a sealed plastic bag. Label and date your mix—it'll keep for weeks!

DONUT PEACH ORCHARD OATMEAL

Serves 4/serving size: 1 1/4 cups

What a way to start the day! Sweet, surprising, and aromatic, this oatmeal belongs in your repertoire of favorite breakfast bowls from spring to fall.

- 2 cups organic unsweetened apple juice
- 1 cup spring water
- 1 1/2 tsp ground cinnamon
- 1/2 tsp sea salt
- 2 cups old-fashioned oats
- 1 (6-oz) container organic fat-free French vanilla yogurt
- 3 fresh donut peaches or 2 medium peaches, chopped (about 1 1/2 cups chopped)
- 2 Tbsp sliced almonds

DIRECTIONS

1. In a medium saucepan, bring the apple juice, water, cinnamon, and salt to a boil over high heat.

2. Stir in the oats and return to a boil. Reduce the heat to medium low and cook 5 minutes, stirring occasionally.

3. Stir in the yogurt and peaches. Continue cooking, stirring occasionally, for 2 minutes or until the oatmeal mixture is heated through. Serve topped with sliced almonds.

Exchanges: 2 starch, 1 1/2 fruit, 1/2 fat; 280 calories, 36 calories from fat, 4 g total fat, 1 g saturated fat, 0 mg cholesterol, 320 mg sodium, 55 g total carbohydrate, 6 g dietary fiber, 22 g sugars, 9 g protein.

FRESH FACT

Peaches are at their seasonal best from May to October, including the squatty-shaped, exceptionally sweet donut peach. Leave the skin on for more fiber. In the winter, frozen organic peaches are a fine find, too. Though usually peeled, frozen peaches and other fruits are generally packed at their peak of ripeness, nutritional value, and flavor. Use a 10-oz bag of frozen peach slices to make 1 1/2 cups chopped.

FOOD FLAIR

You'll notice that any time I call for 1 cup or more of water I specify "spring" water. That's because it just plain tastes better than most tap water, and you'll notice the difference in soups, stews, and beverages. I like to use the same water in cooking I would drink by itself. It's similar to how using decent wine in cooking is preferable to using any ol'cheap one. By paying attention to the quality of every ingredient, you'll enjoy a big flavor difference in the long run.

BLANCO HUEVOS RANCHEROS

Serves 2/serving size: 2 topped tortillas

Though egg yolks are filled with good nutrition, using all egg whites here helps me include other delicious and nutritious fat-containing ingredients—avocado and cheese. It's a Mexican-inspired recipe keeper for breakfast or brunch.

- 4 (5-inch) corn tortillas
- 8 large egg whites or 1 cup 100% egg white substitute
- 1/8 tsp sea salt, or to taste
- 1/4 tsp freshly ground white or black pepper, or to taste

- 3 Tbsp shredded pepper Jack cheese
- 1/2 Hass avocado, peeled and diced (about 1/2 cup)
- 1/4 cup commercially made tomatillo sauce (salsa verde), or see recipe, page 72

- 1/4 cup plain fat-free Greek yogurt, yogurt cheese (see recipe, page 63), or organic low-fat sour cream
- 1 small jalapeño pepper without seeds, minced
- 1 Tbsp chopped fresh cilantro

DIRECTIONS

1. Preheat the oven to 475°F. Lightly coat both sides of the corn tortillas with natural butter-flavored cooking spray and place on a baking sheet. Bake 4 minutes per side or until crisp and lightly browned. Remove from the oven and let cool on the baking sheet.

2. Meanwhile, place a large nonstick skillet over medium heat. Add the egg whites and scramble for 5 minutes or until done. Immediately stir in salt, pepper, and cheese.

3. Place a scoop of cheesy egg whites on top of each crisp tortilla. Top each with avocado, tomatillo sauce, yogurt, jalapeño, and cilantro.

Exchanges: 2 starch, 2 lean meat, 1/2 fat; 300 calories, 93 calories from fat, 10 g total fat, 2 g saturated fat, 5 mg cholesterol, 560 mg sodium, 30 g total carbohydrate, 5 g dietary fiber, 3 g sugars, 21 g protein.

FOOD FLAIR

The seeds and white ribs inside the jalapeño deliver all the heat. Use the seeds in this dish if you like an extra "kick" in the morning. Depending on your skin sensitivity, you might consider wearing protective plastic or rubber gloves when handling the seeds.

MORE THAN FOUR?

This recipe is an impressive morning meal for company. Luckily, it can be easily doubled for 4, tripled for 6, or quadrupled for 8. Just use an extra-large pan for scrambling the egg whites. Also, have all other ingredients prepped and lined up to top the tortillas once the egg whites are scrambled and still hot. If the avocado starts turning brown in the meantime, toss it with the tomatillo sauce.

HEIRLOOM CAPRESE OMELET

Serves 4/serving size: 1/2 omelet

Enjoy a little taste of Italy right in your own home. It'll be a transporting experience when you make this with any variety of heirloom tomatoes picked up fresh at your local farmers' market. But if you can't find heirloom, go for vine-ripened tomatoes, which are usually at their peak in late summer.

- 10 large egg whites or 1 1/4 cups 100% egg white substitute
- 2 large eggs
- 1 Tbsp water
- 1/2 tsp sea salt, or to taste
- 1/4 tsp freshly ground black pepper, or to taste
- 2 tsp extra virgin olive oil (divided use)
- 1 large garlic clove, minced (divided use)
- 1/3 cup shredded part-skim mozzarella cheese (divided use)
- 1 large heirloom or vine-ripened tomato, cut into 12 thin slices
- 12 large fresh basil leaves
- 1 1/2 tsp aged balsamic vinegar, or to taste

DIRECTIONS

1. In a medium bowl, whisk together the egg whites, eggs, water, salt, and pepper until well combined.

2. Heat 1 tsp oil in a large nonstick skillet over medium heat. Sauté half the garlic for 1 minute or until the garlic is fragrant (but don't let it brown). Pour in half the egg mixture.

3. Using a spatula, lift the edges of the eggs as they cook for about 4 minutes, letting the uncooked part run underneath until the omelet is set and the bottom is lightly browned. Sprinkle with half the cheese. Slide out onto a platter, folding omelet over. Slice in half and cover with foil to keep warm.

4. Repeat the process with the remaining oil, garlic, egg mixture, and cheese.

5. Top each omelet half with 3 tomato slices and 3 basil leaves. Drizzle with vinegar to serve.

Exchanges: 1 vegetable, 2 lean meat; 140 calories, 63 calories from fat, 7 g total fat, 2 g saturated fat, 105 mg cholesterol, 500 mg sodium, 4 g total carbohydrate, 1 g dietary fiber, 2 g sugars, 15 g protein.

FRESH FACT !

Once you bring tomatoes home, keep them on the counter, not in the refrigerator. Refrigerating unripe tomatoes adversely affects their texture and flavor.

SAUSAGE–SPINACH SCRAMBLE WITH CARAMELIZED ONIONS

Serves 4/serving size: 1 cup

The balance of flavors in this breakfast dish will have you scrambling for it regularly. And don't worry if the amount of onion seems like a lot. The large amount cooks down to a little—and is exceptionally sweet when caramelized.

- 1 tsp extra virgin olive oil
- 2 3/4 cups very thinly sliced Vidalia, Maui, or other sweet onion
- 1 large garlic clove, minced
- 8 frozen vegetarian breakfast sausage links, cut crosswise into 1/8-inch slices (6 1/2 oz total)
- 6 large egg whites or 3/4 cup 100% egg white substitute
- 1 large egg
- 1/8 tsp sea salt, or to taste
- 1/4 tsp freshly ground black pepper, or to taste
- 1 (5-oz) package organic baby spinach (about 5 cups)
- 1 Tbsp freshly grated Parmigiana-Reggiano cheese

DIRECTIONS

1. Heat the oil in a large nonstick skillet over medium heat. Sauté the onion for 15 minutes or until a rich golden brown, stirring occasionally. Add the garlic and sausage and cook, stirring constantly, for 3 minutes or until the sausage is cooked through.

2. Meanwhile, in a medium bowl, whisk together the egg whites, egg, salt, and pepper.

3. Pour the eggs onto the caramelized onion-sausage mixture in the skillet and scramble for 3 minutes or until done. Remove from heat.

FRESH FACT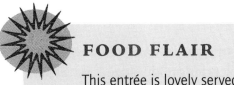

Spinach and egg yolks—two ingredients in this morning meal—both have lutein and zeathan-thin, two antioxidants that may help protect against age-related macular degeneration, the leading cause of irreversible blindness in Americans over age 65.

4. Stir in the spinach until just wilted. (If the pan is not big enough to hold the spinach, combine everything in a large bowl, then quickly reheat in the skillet.) Sprinkle cheese on top of each serving and serve immediately.

Exchanges: 1 carbohydrate, 2 lean meat; 170 calories, 53 calories from fat, 6 g total fat, 1 g saturated fat, 55 mg cholesterol, 580 mg sodium, 16 g total carbohydrate, 4 g dietary fiber, 6 g sugars, 17 g protein.

FOOD FLAIR

This entrée is lovely served with lemon wedges. Each person can squirt to taste for added zing.

FAST FIX

You can slice the onions the day before and refrigerate in a covered container. And you can slice the sausage while frozen and refreeze immediately in a sealed plastic freezer bag. Both will be ready to go in the morning.

DR. SEUSS-INSPIRED GREEN EGGS AND HAM

Serves 4/serving size: 1/2 cup eggs plus 1/2 oz ham

Go ahead ... have some fun with your food! It doesn't get much more fun than eating cartoon-like green food. Not only a kid-pleaser, it's an entire family-pleaser.

- 2 (2-oz) thick slices natural, lean, baked or smoked ham or turkey ham, each cut in half
- 1 large garlic clove
- 1/2 cup loosely packed fresh basil leaves
- 1/4 cup loosely packed fresh flat-leaf parsley leaves
- 6 large egg whites or 3/4 cup 100% egg white substitute
- 2 large eggs
- 2 tsp extra virgin olive oil
- 2 tsp fresh lemon juice
- 1/2 tsp unsalted butter

DIRECTIONS

1. Preheat the oven to 275°F. Wrap the ham in foil and warm in the oven up to 15 minutes.

2. Meanwhile, puree the garlic, basil, parsley, egg whites, eggs, oil, and lemon juice in a blender on low speed for 1 minute or until the egg mixture is an even light green color.

FAST FIX

Blend the green egg mixture the night before you need it. Store it refrigerated in a covered container. Shake the container before scrambling. Also, quickly pan-grill or warm the ham in the microwave instead of the oven.

3. Lightly coat a large nonstick skillet with natural butter-flavored cooking spray. Place over medium heat and melt the butter in the skillet. Add eggs and scramble for 3 minutes or until the eggs are done. Serve eggs with a warm ham slice. Garnish with fresh basil or parsley sprigs, if desired.

Exchanges: 2 lean meat; 120 calories, 55 calories from fat, 6 g total fat, 1 g saturated fat, 125 mg cholesterol, 420 mg sodium, 2 g total carbohydrate, 0 g dietary fiber, 1 g sugars, 13 g protein.

FROTHY SUNRISE YOGURT SMOOTHIE

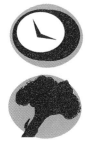

Serves 4/serving size: 1 1/4 cups

This super smoothie tastes like an orange creamsicle in a glass. It's so good you might want to drink it for dessert, not as part of a balanced breakfast.

- 4 large ice cubes (vary quantity depending on desired consistency)
- 2 (6-oz) containers organic low-fat vanilla yogurt
- 1 cup fresh orange juice with pulp
- 3/4 cup organic low-fat milk

DIRECTIONS

Blend all ingredients together on low speed for 30 seconds or until smooth. (If your blender has less than a 5-cup capacity, blend in two even batches.) Serve immediately.

Exchanges: 1/2 fruit, 1 fat-free milk; 120 calories, 15 calories from fat, 2 g total fat, 1 g saturated fat, 5 mg cholesterol, 80 mg sodium, 21 g total carbohydrate, 0 g dietary fiber, 19 g sugars, 6 g protein.

FAST FIX

Combine the yogurt, orange juice, and milk in an opaque beverage container up to 12 hours in advance. Cover and refrigerate. Then just add ice and blend in the morning. By the way, always store orange juice in an opaque container—vitamin C is fragile and can be lost when exposed to too much light, air, or heat.

FOOD FLAIR

For an elegant presentation, serve this gorgeous smoothie in a white wine glass with an orange slice on the rim.

EGGS BENEDICT WITH SILKEN HOLLANDAISE SAUCE

Serves 6/serving size: 1 topped muffin half

There are some rich foods that aren't easily made over into flavor-ful, healthful choices. Thankfully, Eggs Benedict is one that's done here successfully—and succulently. The silken tofu gives the sauce a velvety mouth feel that's unmatched. Plus, the sauce is so peppy you may never go back to regular Hollandaise sauce.

- 4 oz soft silken tofu, undrained (1/2 cup)
- 2 Tbsp fresh lemon juice
- 2 Tbsp fat-free evaporated milk
- 1 tsp unsalted butter
- 2 tsp organic Dijon mustard
- 1 tsp Worcestershire sauce
- 1/8 tsp ground cayenne red pepper, or to taste (optional)
- 3 whole grain or wheat English muffins, halved and toasted
- 6 (1/2-oz) thin slices natural, lean, baked or smoked ham, dry pan-grilled or oven-heated
- 6 medium eggs, poached (see Fresh Fact)

DIRECTIONS

1. Puree the tofu, lemon juice, evaporated milk, butter, mustard, Worcestershire sauce, and red pepper (if using) in a blender on low speed for 30 seconds or until smooth.

2. Place the mixture in a small saucepan over medium-low heat. Simmer for 5 minutes or until hot.

3. Meanwhile, top each toasted muffin half with ham, then a poached egg. Top each with about 3 Tbsp hot Hollandaise sauce to serve.

Exchanges: 1 starch, 1 medium-fat meat, 1/2 fat; 170 calories, 58 calories from fat, 7 g total fat, 2 g saturated fat, 195 mg cholesterol, 490 mg sodium, 16 g total carbohydrate, 2 g dietary fiber, 4 g sugars, 12 g protein.

FRESH FACT

To poach eggs, bring about 3 inches of water to boil in a large (12-inch) shallow sauté pan over high heat. Turn off the heat and add eggs at once by breaking them directly into the water. Immediately cover pan with a tight-fitting lid to retain heat. Allow eggs to cook undisturbed for 4 minutes, or until done as desired. Remove eggs with a perforated spatula or large slotted spoon and drain on plain paper towels.

FOOD FLAIR

Garnish with fresh flat-leaf parsley. Or, if you like extra pep, sprinkle with ground cayenne red pepper.

BAJA BAKED EGG WHITES IN TOMATO CUPS

Serves 2/serving size: 2 cups

Enjoying the natural flavors of good nutrition is easy with these clever "cups." This eye-opening entrée, where the cups are actually tomatoes, will impress a significant other—and you.

- 4 medium, firm, vine-ripened tomatoes
- 4 large egg whites or 1/2 cup 100% egg white substitute
- 1/4 cup salsa (medium heat)
- 1/2 Hass avocado, peeled and cut crosswise into 12 slices
- 1 Tbsp lime juice, or to taste
- 2 Tbsp chopped fresh cilantro

DIRECTIONS

1. Preheat the oven to 450°F. Slice about 3/4 inch off the top of each tomato. With a spoon, scoop out the insides of each tomato to form tomato cups; reserve insides for another use.

2. Place tomato cups on a nonstick pan, or place each into a ramekin or small, round baking dish. Add 1 egg white to each cup and top with 1 Tbsp salsa.

3. Bake for 25 minutes or until the egg whites are firm. Remove from the oven and top each cup with 3 avocado slices arranged like a fan. Drizzle with lime juice and top with cilantro.

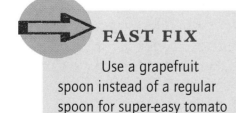

FAST FIX

Use a grapefruit spoon instead of a regular spoon for super-easy tomato scooping.

Exchanges: 1 carbohydrate, 1 lean meat, 1/2 fat; 160 calories, 65 calories from fat, 7 g total fat, 1 g saturated fat, 0 mg cholesterol, 310 mg sodium, 16 g total carbohydrate, 4 g dietary fiber, 9 g sugars, 10 g protein.

FRESH FACT

If you're using fresh tomatoes and avocados that are perfectly ripe, they're so wonderful that no added salt or pepper should be required to make this dish more flavorful. Plus, lime juice acts a bit like salt in flavoring the avocados. Also, if the best tomatoes you find are small or large, adjust the amount of egg whites accordingly. The tomato cup should be about 3/4 full of egg white before you add the salsa.

FOOD FLAIR

Finely dice the reserved tomato tops and use as a garnish. For added nutrition and flavor, add the scooped out tomato pulp to soup, stews, or the simmering liquid of brown rice or other whole grains.

GRANNY SMITH BREAKFAST SAUSAGE PATTIES

Serves 4/serving size: 2 patties

These substantial patties are best served two at a time for a morning entrée. They can be served singly as a side dish, too. They're a cross between sausage patties and burgers. And the wholesome apples and oats make these patties well balanced and deliciously moist.

- 1/2 lb ground chicken breast (antibiotic free)
- 1/4 lb lean ground beef sirloin (antibiotic free)
- 1 medium Granny Smith apple, cored, peeled, and coarsely grated
- 2 (1-oz) packets organic instant oatmeal (about 2/3 cup total)
- 1/4 cup coarsely grated red onion
- 1/4 cup chopped fresh flat-leaf parsley
- 1 Tbsp finely chopped fresh sage (about 6 large leaves)
- 1 tsp minced fresh rosemary (optional)
- 3/4 tsp sea salt, or to taste
- 1/2 tsp freshly ground black pepper, or to taste
- 1 large egg, lightly beaten

DIRECTIONS

1. In a large bowl, combine all ingredients with your hands. Form the mixture into 8 patties (use about 1/3 cup mixture for each patty).

2. Place a large nonstick skillet over medium heat. Cook patties in batches 4 minutes per side or until well done, turning over once. Remove cooked patties to a plate and keep covered with foil until all the patties are done.

Exchanges: 1 carbohydrate, 2 lean meat; 200 calories, 46 calories from fat, 5 g total fat, 1 g saturated fat, 95 mg cholesterol, 530 mg sodium, 17 g total carbohydrate, 2 g dietary fiber, 5 g sugars, 21 g protein.

FAST FIX

You can form the patties at night, cover with plastic wrap, refrigerate, then cook in the morning. Cook the chilled patties for 5 minutes per side or until well done.

MORE THAN FOUR?

Prepare 16 mini patties with this recipe.
Cook 3 to 4 minutes per side or until well done.
Serve 2 to each person as a side dish
for breakfast or brunch.

GARLIC-SPIKED HOMESTYLE HASH BROWNS

Serves 6/serving size: 2/3 cup

Your taste buds will get a wakeup call from these kicked-up hash browns. They're so tasty you'll think they're full of fat. Lucky for you, they're not. But the fat this side dish does have helps reduce the glycemic effect of the potatoes—so they won't cause a dramatic blood glucose spike.

- 1 Tbsp extra virgin olive oil
- 2 tsp unsalted butter (divided use)
- 1 cup chopped red onion
- 2 large garlic cloves, minced
- 3 medium Yukon gold or red potatoes, boiled with peel, chilled and diced (1/2-inch cubes; about 4 cups)
- 3/4 tsp sea salt, or to taste
- 1/4 tsp ground cayenne red pepper, or to taste
- 1/4 cup roughly chopped fresh Italian parsley
- 2 Tbsp finely chopped fresh chives

DIRECTIONS

1. Heat the oil and 1 tsp butter in a large nonstick skillet over medium-high heat. Sauté the onion for 3 minutes, then add garlic and sauté for 1 minute.

2. Add the potatoes and cook for 5 minutes or until potatoes are lightly browned, turning occasionally. Remove from heat and stir in the remaining butter. Sprinkle evenly with salt and red pepper. Stir in parsley and chives.

Exchanges: 1 1/2 starch, 1/2 fat; 120 calories, 33 calories from fat, 4 g total fat, 1 g saturated fat, 5 mg cholesterol, 300 mg sodium, 19 g total carbohydrate, 2 g dietary fiber, 1 g sugars, 3 g protein.

FAST FIX

Boil the potatoes until they're just cooked through, yet still somewhat firm. Be careful not to overcook them—you'll wind up with mushy hash browns. Refrigerate cooked potatoes in a sealed container for up to 2 days.

FRESH FACT

Potatoes are packed with more antioxidants than you'd think . . . and when you enjoy the peel, the fiber is a healthful added bonus.

NATURAL ALMOND BUTTER AND BANANA TOASTIE

Serves 4/serving size: 1 toastie

Peanut butter 'n' jelly is a favorite—for kids and adults. But now there's a better way to do it—toasted with almond butter instead of peanut and fresh banana instead of sugary jelly. Perhaps it'll become your new favorite!

- 7 Tbsp natural unsalted almond butter
- 8 (1 1/4-oz) slices whole grain bread
- 2 1/2 large fully ripened bananas, gently mashed or thinly sliced (about 1 1/4 cups)

DIRECTIONS

1. Spread the almond butter on 4 bread slices and top with mashed banana. Top with remaining bread slices. Spray the sandwich with natural butter-flavored cooking spray.

2. Place each sandwich on a preheated panini press (cook in batches, if necessary). Lightly place the panini top on the sandwiches and grill 5 minutes or until toasted.

3. Alternatively, pan-toast each sandwich in a preheated nonstick skillet over medium-high heat for 2 minutes on the first side and 1 minute on the other side, or until toasted.

4. Slice Toasties in half diagonally and serve immediately.

Exchanges: 2 1/2 starch, 1 fruit, 3 1/2 fat; 420 calories, 174 calories from fat, 19 g total fat, 2 g saturated fat, 0 mg cholesterol, 320 mg sodium, 56 g total carbohydrate, 7 g dietary fiber, 17 g sugars, 12 g protein.

FOOD FLAIR

You'll love a panini press. It's ideal for grilling both sides of just about any sandwich (think: gooey grilled cheese!) at the same time. You can grill beef, chicken, fish, or veggies on it, too. Perhaps the best part . . . it makes those lovely grill marks.

FAST FIX

Prepare sandwiches (untoasted) up to several hours in advance (or overnight), cover, and refrigerate. Grill or pan-toast just before serving.

FRESH FACT

Many studies have shown that regular nut consumption may protect against risk of diabetes and heart disease. Also, almonds and almond butter help provide satiety—the feeling of fullness—so eating them may ultimately help you stick to your meal plan.

BANANA BREAD SQUARES

Serves 16/serving size: 1 square

When I was growing up, my mother baked banana bread, froze it, and sliced it into paper-thin slices for my after-school snack. I thought it was such a treat—like having dessert before dinner. Here, I've updated her recipe. It's now perfect for a little breakfast bite, too . . . just grab a square and go!

- 2 Tbsp unsalted butter, melted
- 2 Tbsp canola oil
- 2/3 cup turbinado sugar
- 3 egg whites or 6 Tbsp 100% egg white substitute
- 3 large extra-ripe bananas, mashed (about 1 1/3 cups)
- 1 1/2 tsp pure vanilla extract
- 3/4 cup unbleached all-purpose flour
- 3/4 cup finely ground whole wheat flour
- 1 tsp baking soda
- 1/4 tsp sea salt
- 1/4 cup chopped walnuts (optional)

DIRECTIONS

1. Preheat the oven to 350°F. Lightly coat an 8 × 8-inch nonstick cake pan with natural cooking spray.

2. In a large mixing bowl, whisk together the melted butter, oil, and sugar. Add the egg whites and whisk until well combined. Add the mashed bananas and vanilla extract and whisk until well combined.

3. In a separate bowl, sift together the flours, baking soda, and salt. (If you don't have a sifter, just shake all ingredients through a mesh strainer.) Add to the banana mixture and stir until just combined. Pour the batter into the pan. Sprinkle, then very lightly press the walnuts (if using) onto the batter.

4. Bake for 30 to 35 minutes or until springy to the touch. Cool on a rack, then slice into squares. This tastes great semi-frozen, too.

Exchanges: 1 carbohydrate, 1/2 fat; 110 calories, 29 calories from fat, 3 g total fat, 1 g saturated fat, 5 mg cholesterol, 125 mg sodium, 17 g total carbohydrate, 1 g dietary fiber, 8 g sugars, 2 g protein.

FRESH FACT

Turbinado sugar is a slightly coarser, more natural alternative to regular granulated white sugar, which is further processed. Turbinado is made from the first pressing of the sugar cane, which leaves it with a light, crystal-like brown color, and a wonderful flavor from its natural molasses. In cooking and baking, use the same amount of turbinado sugar as granulated white sugar in a recipe—1 cup for 1 cup.

HOMEMADE GRANOLA— RASPBERRY PARFAITS

Serves 4/serving size: 1 parfait

Vegetarians (and non-vegetarians) rejoice! Fiber never tasted so good. This scrumptious parfait makes a picture-perfect meal-in-one!

- 1 1/2 cups old-fashioned oats
- 1/3 cup slivered almonds
- 3 Tbsp raw wheat germ
- 2 Tbsp shelled sunflower seeds, unsalted
- 2 tsp ground cinnamon
- 2 Tbsp natural unsweetened apple butter
- 2 Tbsp acacia or other mild floral honey
- 2 (6-oz) containers raspberry or vanilla soy yogurt
- 1 1/3 cups fresh raspberries

DIRECTIONS

1. Preheat the oven to 325°F. In a medium bowl, stir together the oats, almonds, wheat germ, sunflower seeds, and cinnamon.

2. In a small bowl, stir together the apple butter and honey. Add to the oat mixture and stir until thoroughly combined.

3. Spread the mixture evenly on a large baking pan. Bake for 25 minutes or until toasted and nearly crisp, stirring occasionally. Remove from the oven and let cool slightly to further crisp.

4. Layer the granola, yogurt, and berries into each parfait, wine, or other large beverage glass.

FAST FIX

You can prepare this granola ahead of time and store in an airtight container at room temperature for several days. And if you're super time-crunched, try this parfait with your favorite brand of natural granola.

Exchanges: 4 carbohydrate, 1 fat; 350 calories, 93 calories from fat, 10 g total fat, 1 g saturated fat, 0 mg cholesterol, 15 mg sodium, 59 g total carbohydrate, 9 g dietary fiber, 25 g sugars, 11 g protein.

HIP DIPS

CARIBBEAN BLACK BEAN DIP

Serves 8/serving size: 3 1/2 Tbsp

Canned beans can be tasty—and time-saving. But go with the organic canned varieties for the freshest flavors. In this sublime dip, the combination of beans and avocado creates a velvety texture.

- 1 (15.5-oz) can organic black beans, drained
- 1/2 Hass avocado, peeled and sliced
- 3 Tbsp lemon juice
- 2 Tbsp roughly chopped cilantro
- 1/4 tsp ground cayenne red pepper
- 1/4 tsp ground cumin
- 1/4 tsp sea salt, or to taste
- 3 Tbsp thinly sliced green onion

DIRECTIONS

Puree all ingredients except the green onion in a blender until smooth. Top with green onion and serve in a bowl with tortilla chips.

Exchanges: 1/2 carbohydrate, 1/2 fat; 60 calories, 15 calories from fat, 2 g total fat, 0 g saturated fat, 0 mg cholesterol, 125 mg sodium, 9 g total carbohydrate, 3 g dietary fiber, 2 g sugars, 3 g protein.

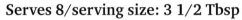

FOOD FLAIR

For best results, refrigerate this creamy dip at least 30 minutes prior to serving. You might find it better the next day! And for added flavor, stir in 1/8 tsp freshly ground nutmeg.

FAST FIX

Create a spice mixture. In a small jar or sealable plastic bag, add 1 Tbsp each ground cayenne red pepper, ground cumin, and sea salt. Label it "Caribbean Spice Mix." Use 3/4 tsp of this mixture whenever you make this dip. Enjoy it as a spice rub for meat, poultry, or fish, too.

JALAPEÑO–PEANUT HUMMUS WITH FRESH HERBS

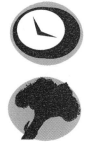

Serves 6/serving size: 1/4 cup

Use natural peanut butter instead of the traditional tahini (sesame paste) to create a trendy, tasty version of this Middle Eastern-style dip.

- 1 (15-oz) can organic chickpeas (garbanzo beans), drained
- 1 small jalapeño pepper, with or without seeds
- 1 large garlic clove
- 1 Tbsp natural creamy peanut butter
- 2 Tbsp lemon juice
- 1/4 cup water
- 1/4 tsp sea salt, or to taste
- 3 Tbsp chopped fresh cilantro or flat-leaf parsley

DIRECTIONS

Puree all ingredients except the cilantro in a blender until smooth, adding more water by tablespoonfuls only if necessary. Top with or stir in cilantro and serve with raw vegetables or fresh whole wheat pita wedges.

Exchanges: 1/2 carbohydrate, 1/2 fat; 60 calories, 15 calories from fat, 2 g total fat, 0 g saturated fat, 0 mg cholesterol, 105 mg sodium, 9 g total carbohydrate, 2 g dietary fiber, 1 g sugars, 3 g protein.

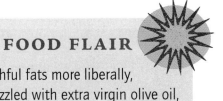

FOOD FLAIR

For those who can enjoy healthful fats more liberally, serve this zesty hummus drizzled with extra virgin olive oil, then topped with fresh flat-leaf parsley.

MEXICALI LAYER DIP

Serves 16/serving size: 1/2 cup

This is a fantastically bold dip sure to satisfy everyone at your next big gathering. It's a real party-pleaser.

- 1 (16-oz) can natural fat-free vegetarian refried beans
- 1/2 tsp hot pepper sauce, or to taste
- 1 1/2 cups freshly prepared store-bought guacamole
- 3/4 cup organic low-fat sour cream
- 2 Tbsp lime juice (divided use)
- 3/4 tsp chili powder
- 2 medium vine-ripened tomatoes, seeded and diced (1 1/2 cups)
- 1 cup thinly sliced green onion
- 3/4 cup shredded Mexican-style cheese or Monterey Jack cheese

DIRECTIONS

1. In a small bowl, combine the refried beans and hot pepper sauce. Spread on a large platter or in a 9 × 13-inch clear glass baking dish. Thinly spread the guacamole on top of the beans.

2. In another bowl, combine the sour cream, 1 Tbsp lime juice, and chili powder. Spread the mixture evenly on top of the guacamole layer.

3. Toss the tomatoes with the remaining lime juice in another small bowl. Sprinkle the tomatoes, green onion, and cheese on the sour cream layer. Serve chilled with baked blue corn tortilla chips.

Exchanges: 1/2 carbohydrate, 1/2 fat; 70 calories, 29 calories from fat, 3 g total fat, 1 g saturated fat, 5 mg cholesterol, 135 mg sodium, 6 g total carbohydrate, 2 g dietary fiber, 1 g sugars, 3 g protein.

FRESH FACT

If you'd like to make your own guacamole instead of using store-bought, try Classic Guacamole (see recipe, page 68).

FOOD FLAIR

If you choose to serve this as a warm instead of chilled dip, prepare it without the guacamole layer. Serve the cool guacamole on the side.

FAST FIX

Instead of combining refried beans and hot pepper sauce, simply use spicy refried beans. Just be sure to use a natural or organic variety.

MINTED ENGLISH CUCUMBER TZATZIKI DIP

Serves 8/serving size: 1/4 cup

Traditionally, you might find Tzatziki served as a sauce for a Greek gyro. But it's much more versatile than you might realize. Serve it as a veggie or chip dip, a condiment for meats, or a sauce for sandwiches. And now it's easier than ever to fix, since fat-free Greek yogurt is now readily available.

- 1 Tbsp extra virgin olive oil
- 2 Tbsp lemon juice
- 2 large garlic cloves, minced
- 1 cup plain fat-free Greek yogurt or yogurt cheese (see Fresh Fact)
- 1/4 tsp sea salt, or to taste
- 1/8 tsp freshly ground black pepper, or to taste
- 1 1/8 cups finely diced English (hothouse) cucumber with skin
- 2 Tbsp finely chopped fresh mint
- 1 Tbsp minced fresh dill

DIRECTIONS

1. In a medium bowl, vigorously stir the olive oil, lemon juice, garlic, yogurt, salt, and pepper together. Stir in the cucumber, mint, and dill. Cover and refrigerate until chilled.

2. Serve with stuffed grape leaves or grilled or roasted meat or poultry—with pita on the side. Or serve as a dip with whole wheat pita wedges. The dip tastes great for days!

Exchanges: 1 carbohydrate, 1/2 fat; 100 calories, 32 calories from fat, 4 g total fat, 0 g saturated fat, 5 mg cholesterol, 220 mg sodium, 13 g total carbohydrate, 0 g dietary fiber, 8 g sugars, 6 g protein.

FRESH FACT

To make your own yogurt cheese (it's basically Greek yogurt!), line a mesh strainer with cheesecloth or a double layer of plain paper towels. Place 18 oz (or three 6-oz containers) plain fat-free yogurt in the lined strainer. Place the strainer over a bowl and allow the yogurt to drain, refrigerated, at least 4 hours or overnight. Makes 1 rounded cup.

FOOD FLAIR

For those who can enjoy healthful fats more liberally, double the extra virgin olive oil in this Mediterranean-inspired dip.

ZESTY ORANGE–GINGER DIP

Serves 10/serving size: 2 Tbsp

The secret to this dip is its tanginess and tartness. It works its magic best with savory dishes. Taste its special power by pairing it with Asian-Style Pork Meatballs (see recipe, page 87) or Chili–Lime Crisped Chicken Fingers (see recipe, page 90).

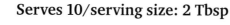

- 1 cup plain low-fat yogurt
- 1/2 tsp toasted sesame oil
- 3 Tbsp freshly squeezed orange juice
- 2 tsp grated fresh ginger
- 1/2 tsp orange zest (grated peel)

DIRECTIONS

In a medium bowl, whisk the yogurt and oil until well combined. Whisk in the juice, ginger, and zest.

Exchanges: free; 20 calories, 6 calories from fat, 1 g total fat, 0 g saturated fat, 0 mg cholesterol, 15 mg sodium, 2 g total carbohydrate, 0 g dietary fiber, 2 g sugars, 1 g protein.

FOOD FLAIR

Dips can often double as condiments. Spread this cool condiment onto chicken, pork, or turkey sandwiches.

HIPSTER HERB DIP

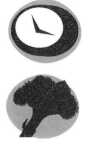

Serves 12/serving size: scant 3 Tbsp

It's practically a must to have raw veggies and dip available at any big gathering—but next time, serve a real dip that everyone can enjoy freely. This full-flavored dip has fat . . . but it's low in saturated fat and has no trans fat. And, with vegetables, the percentage of fat that you actually get is well within a healthful range.

- 1 cup organic low-fat cottage cheese
- 1/2 cup organic low-fat sour cream
- 1/4 cup mayonnaise

- 2 large garlic cloves, minced
- 1 large shallot, minced
- 1/4 cup finely chopped fresh flat-leaf parsley
- 1/4 cup minced fresh chives

- 1/2 tsp Worcestershire sauce
- 1/4 tsp sea salt, or to taste
- 1/4 tsp hot pepper sauce, or to taste

DIRECTIONS
Stir all ingredients together in a large bowl.

Exchanges: 1 1/2 fat; 70 calories, 43 calories from fat, 5 g total fat, 1 g saturated fat, 5 mg cholesterol, 135 mg sodium, 2 g total carbohydrate, 0 g dietary fiber, 1 g sugars, 3 g protein.

FOOD FLAIR
For best results, refrigerate this dip at least 1 hour prior to serving. And for added flavor interest, stir in 1/8 tsp freshly grated or ground nutmeg before serving.

MORE THAN FOUR
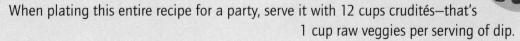
When plating this entire recipe for a party, serve it with 12 cups crudités—that's 1 cup raw veggies per serving of dip.

SPA SPINACH DIP

Serves 20/serving size: 2 1/2 Tbsp

It's likely you've only had spinach dip made with a package of vegetable soup mix. Though full of flavor, it's also loaded with artificial ingredients. It's full of sodium and fat, too. Now you can finally savor this popular party dip with 100% real ingredients and fresh flavor that will astound you.

- 1 (10-oz) package frozen chopped organic spinach, thawed
- 1 cup organic low-fat sour cream
- 1/2 cup mayonnaise

- 1 (8-oz) can water chestnuts, drained and thinly sliced
- 3/4 cup thinly sliced green onion
- 1/4 cup grated carrots
- 1 large garlic clove, minced

- 3/4 tsp sea salt, or to taste
- 1/4 tsp hot pepper sauce, or to taste
- 1/8 tsp freshly grated or ground nutmeg, or to taste

DIRECTIONS

1. Over a small bowl, squeeze the spinach in a double layer of plain paper towels until thoroughly dry. Reserve the liquid for another purpose, such as making soup or rice.

2. Combine all ingredients in a medium bowl. Serve chilled with pumpernickel or rye bread pieces, or use as a dip for veggies.

Exchanges: 1 1/2 fat; 70 calories, 50 calories from fat, 6 g total fat, 1 g saturated fat, 5 mg cholesterol, 150 mg sodium, 2 g total carbohydrate, 1 g dietary fiber, 1 g sugars, 1 g protein.

FRESH FACT

Dips are definitely fun—making them a perfect party food. However, they're also ideal for parties since you can make most of them, including this spinach dip, in advance. Dips made in advance are usually tastier, too, because all the flavors have blended. So make this recipe 1 day before a special gathering—and keep chilled until you're ready to serve.

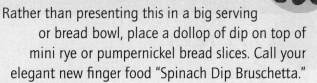

MORE THAN FOUR?

Rather than presenting this in a big serving or bread bowl, place a dollop of dip on top of mini rye or pumpernickel bread slices. Call your elegant new finger food "Spinach Dip Bruschetta."

FAST FIX

Purchase bread in a presliced mini loaf. Then there's no need to slice it yourself. Or serve the dip in a hollowed-out loaf of pumpernickel bread. Tear out pieces from the center by hand before you fill the loaf with dip.

CLASSIC GUACAMOLE

Serves 10/serving size: 1/4 cup

There's no need to say "no" to guacamole. The avocados in it are high in the "good" kind of fat—mostly monounsaturated. And since they're fruits, they provide a wealth of heart-protective nutrients, including potassium, vitamin E, and folate. What's more, avocados act like nutrient boosters, helping the body absorb more fat-soluble nutrients from the foods you eat with them. So whatever you enjoy this guacamole with will be better for you, too.

- 2 Hass avocados, peeled and cubed
- 1 Tbsp lime juice, or to taste
- 1 medium vine-ripened tomato, seeded and finely diced (3/4 cup)
- 1/4 cup chopped white onion
- 2 Tbsp chopped fresh cilantro
- 1 small jalapeño pepper with or without seeds, minced
- 1/4 tsp sea salt, or to taste

DIRECTIONS

Gently stir all ingredients together in a medium bowl until just combined. Add additional lime juice and salt to taste (optional). Serve with baked white, yellow, or blue corn tortilla chips.

Exchanges: 1 fat; 60 calories, 49 calories from fat, 5 g total fat, 1 g saturated fat, 0 mg cholesterol, 60 mg sodium, 4 g total carbohydrate, 3 g dietary fiber, 1 g sugars, 1 g protein.

FRESH FACT

Avocados are good for the environment. Like all tree orchards, avocado orchards help keep air fresh by producing oxygen and absorbing carbon dioxide. Just one California avocado tree can absorb the same amount of carbon dioxide each year produced by a car driven about 26,000 miles. A couple of mature avocado trees can provide enough oxygen for an entire family—or your four best friends.

BALSAMIC–BASIL TOFUNNAISE

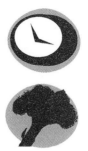

Serves 8/serving size: 1 1/2 Tbsp

It's an earthy, zingy, oh-so-tasty basil "mayo." It's sensational as a condiment for burgers or sandwiches, like Pan-Grilled Veggie Ciabatta (see recipe, page 194). It's especially good with grilled artichoke hearts, too.

- 4 oz soft silken tofu, drained (1/2 cup)
- 2 Tbsp aged balsamic vinegar
- 12 large fresh basil leaves
- 2 Tbsp pine nuts
- 1 large garlic clove

DIRECTIONS

Puree all ingredients in a blender until smooth.

Exchanges: 1/2 fat; 25 calories, 17 calories from fat, 2 g total fat, 0 g saturated fat, 0 mg cholesterol, 0 mg sodium, 1 g total carbohydrate, 0 g dietary fiber, 1 g sugars, 1 g protein.

! FRESH FACT

Silken tofu has a silky smooth texture that provides that creamy mouth feel that's so desirable in dips and smoothies—and in tofunnaises.

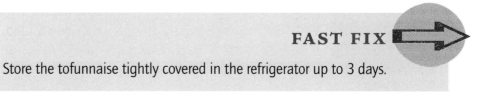

FAST FIX

Store the tofunnaise tightly covered in the refrigerator up to 3 days.

TABLESIDE CALIFORNIA AVOCADO– BLACK MISSION FIG GUACAMOLE

Serves 12/serving size: 3 Tbsp

This chunky guacamole is not any ordinary guacamole. It has figs in it! You might find this fruity, yet spicy, figgy guacamole is better than the original.

- 2 Hass avocados, peeled and cubed
- 3 fresh Black Mission figs, diced, or 2 dried figs, finely diced
- 1/4 cup finely chopped red onion
- 1 small jalapeño pepper with seeds, minced
- 2 Tbsp finely chopped fresh cilantro
- 2 Tbsp lime juice
- 1/8 tsp ground cumin
- 1/2 tsp sea salt, or to taste

FAST FIX

How do you easily prep an avocado? One way is to slice an avocado from top to bottom, all the way around, until you hit the seed. Twist the avocado to form two halves. Hold the seed-containing half in one hand or place it on the counter and firmly, yet carefully, wedge the knife blade into the seed. Twist the knife to remove the seed. With a large spoon, scoop out the avocado as close to the skin as possible.

DIRECTIONS

Gently stir all ingredients together in a medium bowl until just combined. Serve with baked blue corn tortilla chips.

Exchanges: 1/2 carbohydrate, 1 1/2 fat; 90 calories, 61 calories from fat, 7 g total fat, 1 g saturated fat, 0 mg cholesterol, 150 mg sodium, 8 g total carbohydrate, 4 g dietary fiber, 3 g sugars, 1 g protein.

TOMATO—CILANTRO SALSA FRESCA

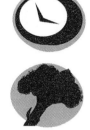

Serves 8/serving size: rounded 1/4 cup

On a Mexican menu, you might see this salsa called "pico de gallo" or "salsa Mexicana." But whatever you decide to call it, the most important thing is to eat it. You might never go back to the jarred variety after enjoying this easy, fresh salsa.

- 2 medium vine-ripened tomatoes, seeded and diced (1 1/2 cups)
- 1 serrano pepper with some seeds, minced
- 1 cup diced white onion
- 1 Tbsp finely chopped fresh cilantro
- 1 Tbsp lime juice
- 1/2 tsp sea salt, or to taste

DIRECTIONS

Combine all ingredients in a medium bowl. Serve with baked white, yellow, or blue corn tortilla chips, or use as a topping for meat, poultry, or fish.

Exchanges: free; 15 calories, 0 calories from fat, 0 g total fat, 0 g saturated fat, 0 mg cholesterol, 150 mg sodium, 3 g total carbohydrate, 1 g dietary fiber, 2 g sugars, 1 g protein.

! FRESH FACT

Salsa is actually the Spanish word for sauce. There are lots of salsas: picante (spicy), verde (green), and fresca (fresh)—just to name a few.

SALSA VERDE

Serves 4/serving size: 1/4 cup

Try this tasty salsa in Blanco Huevos Rancheros (see recipe, page 36) or California Avocado–Bean Salad with Salsa Verde (see recipe, page 144). It's equally delicious with baked tortilla chips. In fact, you might find yourself enjoying this green salsa more often than the traditional red.

- 1/2 lb tomatillos, husks removed and rinsed (6 to 8 tomatillos)
- 1/4 cup loosely packed cilantro leaves
- 1 slice medium white onion
- 1 large garlic clove
- 1/8 tsp sea salt, or to taste
- 1 Tbsp lime juice (optional)

DIRECTIONS

1. Place the whole tomatillos in a large saucepan and fill with water to cover. Bring to a boil over high heat, then reduce heat to low and simmer 10 minutes or until softened.

2. Drain and chop the tomatillos. Puree half of them, along with the cilantro, onion, and garlic, in a blender until smooth.

3. Return the puree to the saucepan and add the remaining chopped tomatillos. Cook over medium-low heat for 5 minutes, stirring occasionally. Add salt and lime juice (if using). Serve at room temperature.

Exchanges: free; 20 calories, 5 calories from fat, 1 g total fat, 0 g saturated fat, 0 mg cholesterol, 75 mg sodium, 4 g total carbohydrate, 1 g dietary fiber, 2 g sugars, 1 g protein.

FRESH FACT

Though tomatillos look like small green tomatoes wrapped in papery husks, they're not tomatoes at all. Rather, these acidic fruits are relatives of gooseberries.

MORE THAN FOUR?

Serve chips along with two kinds of salsa: a red tomato-based one and this green tomatillo-based one. The red and green colors are especially festive in the winter holidays.

FOOD FLAIR

If you serve this salsa alone, such as a dip for chips, squirt in some lime juice before serving. But if you want to add it to another recipe, leave out the lime . . . then adjust the seasonings in the entire dish, not just the salsa.

BELL PEPPER–AVOCADO "CRÈME" SAUCE

Serves 12/serving size: 1/4 cup

Enjoy this antioxidant-rich, vivid orange, velvety smooth sauce along with Sweet Potato Burrito Spirals (see recipe, page 196). Or use it like gravy to add flavor and visual pizzazz to a plate of chicken and rice. Try it as a sandwich spread instead of mayo or mustard, too. It's surprisingly versatile and oh-so-tasty.

- 1 tsp extra virgin olive oil
- 4 cups chopped red bell pepper
- 1 small jalapeño pepper with seeds, chopped
- 3/4 cup chopped red onion
- 1 Hass avocado, peeled and cubed
- 1/4 cup lime juice
- 1/4 tsp sea salt, or to taste

DIRECTIONS

1. Heat the oil in a large nonstick skillet over medium-high heat. Sauté the red peppers, jalapeño, and onion for 12 minutes or until softened, stirring frequently. Remove from heat and let cool slightly.

2. Puree the pepper mixture, avocado, lime juice, and salt in a blender until velvety smooth. (Be patient with the blending process, scraping down sides as needed.) Serve warm or at room temperature.

Exchanges: 1 vegetable, 1/2 fat; 40 calories, 22 calories from fat, 2 g total fat, 0 g saturated fat, 0 mg cholesterol, 50 mg sodium, 5 g total carbohydrate, 2 g dietary fiber, 2 g sugars, 1 g protein.

FAST FIX

Make this sauce in advance and freeze it in a sealed container. Thaw it in the refrigerator the day before you plan to use it. Reheat the sauce in a saucepan over medium-high heat until it begins to bubble.

FOOD FLAIR

For a roasted flavor, cook the peppers and onion over medium-high heat for 5 minutes, then over high heat for 5 minutes. The blackened parts of the peppers will add dark flecks of rich roasted flavor to the sauce. For more spiciness, use a whole, large jalapeño pepper—or just add hot sauce to taste.

SCALLION YOGURT CHEESE

Serves 4/serving size: scant 1/4 cup

Move over, sour cream! Your baked potato has a new calcium-rich, calorie-friendly pal. This yogurt cheese is yummy dolloped on top of a baked potato. It can be used as condiment instead of mayo for a grilled chicken wrap or turkey pita, too.

- 1 3/4 cups fat-free plain yogurt
- 2 Tbsp minced green onion
- 1 small garlic clove, minced
- 1/8 tsp sea salt, or to taste

DIRECTIONS

1. Line a mesh strainer with cheesecloth or a double layer of plain paper towels. Place the yogurt in the strainer. Place the strainer over a bowl and allow it to drain, refrigerated, for at least 4 hours.

2. In a small bowl, whisk the yogurt cheese with green onion, garlic, and salt.

Exchanges: 1/2 fat-free milk; 40 calories, 0 calories from fat, 0 g total fat, 0 g saturated fat, 0 mg cholesterol, 125 mg sodium, 8 g total carbohydrate, 0 g dietary fiber, 5 g sugars, 4 g protein.

FRESH FACT

Inulin (not insulin) is a form of dietary fiber found naturally in onions, garlic, leeks, jicama, and chicory root. It isn't broken down by the body into simple sugars, so it has very little impact on blood glucose levels. Plus, it may play a beneficial role in health, including digestive health. It's frequently added to yogurt, where it provides additional bulk.

FAST FIX

This recipe will take just a few minutes to fix if you use fat-free Greek yogurt in place of the regular yogurt. It'll cost more, but there's no need to strain the yogurt for 4 hours. That's already done for you. Use about 1 cup fat-free Greek yogurt and skip to Step 2.

COOL THAI PEANUT SAUCE

Serves 8/serving size: 2 Tbsp

Though highly flavored, this is a multipurpose sauce. It can be a dipping sauce for chicken fingers or a satay-style sauce with chicken kebabs. It's also delightful tossed with noodles for a cool salad.

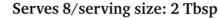

- 1/3 cup rice vinegar
- 1/4 cup natural creamy peanut butter
- 2 Tbsp lime juice

- 1 Tbsp toasted sesame oil
- 1 Tbsp naturally brewed reduced-sodium soy sauce
- 1 Tbsp peeled fresh ginger root

- 1 Tbsp orange blossom or clover honey
- 1 large garlic clove
- 1/4 tsp hot pepper sauce

DIRECTIONS

Puree all ingredients in a blender until smooth. (If you don't have a powerful blender, mince the garlic and grate the ginger root before blending.)

Exchanges: 1/2 carbohydrate, 1 fat; 80 calories, 51 calories from fat, 6 g total fat, 1 g saturated fat, 0 mg cholesterol, 105 mg sodium, 5 g total carbohydrate, 1 g dietary fiber, 3 g sugars, 2 g protein.

FOOD FLAIR

Cook 4 oz soba noodles according to package directions, omitting added oil and salt. Drain well. Toss with 2 tsp toasted sesame oil. Chill, then toss noodles with 1/4 cup of this sauce. This makes 3 servings of 1 scant cup each. Enjoy the noodles as a side dish garnished with fresh cilantro. Jazz it up and serve it as a salad tossed with roasted sesame seeds or finely chopped roasted peanuts, bean sprouts, grated carrots, grated cucumber, and sliced green onion.

SPATIZERS & SMALL PLATES

TROPICAL SHRIMP COCKTAIL

Serves 4/serving size: scant 1 cup

Savor this sexy shrimp cocktail. The lime wedge on the serving glass rim makes it prettier, too.

- 1 lb raw farm-raised large shrimp, shelled, deveined, and tails removed
- 1/2 cup grape tomatoes, quartered
- 1/3 cup diced jicama
- 1/3 cup diced Vidalia, Maui, or other sweet onion
- 1 large jalapeño pepper with or without seeds, minced
- 2 Tbsp chopped fresh cilantro
- 1 recipe Baja Shrimp Cocktail Sauce (see Fresh Fact)
- 1/2 Hass avocado, peeled and diced (about 1/2 cup)
- 1 lime, halved

DIRECTIONS

1. Place a large saucepan filled about 3/4 full of water over high heat and bring to a boil. Plunge the shrimp into the boiling water. Reduce the heat to medium low and cook shrimp for 3 minutes or until opaque and firm. Drain, then immediately place the shrimp in a bowl of ice water to stop the cooking process (or rinse quickly under cold water for 1 to 2 minutes). Drain the shrimp, pat dry, and dice.

2. In a large bowl, gently stir together the shrimp, tomatoes, jicama, onion, jalapeño, cilantro, and sauce.

3. To serve, divide the shrimp cocktail among 4 martini or other glasses or small dishes. Top with avocado and drizzle with juice from one lime half. Cut the other lime half into 4 wedges and place a wedge onto each glass rim. Serve chilled as is or with whole grain corn tortilla chips.

Exchanges: 1/2 carbohydrate, 2 lean meat; 150 calories, 40 calories from fat, 4 g total fat, 1 g saturated fat, 170 mg cholesterol, 360 mg sodium, 10 g total carbohydrate, 3 g dietary fiber, 5 g sugars, 19 g protein.

FRESH FACT

To make Baja Shrimp Cocktail Sauce, combine 3 Tbsp organic ketchup, 1/4 cup vegetable or tomato juice (regular or spicy), 2 Tbsp lime juice, and 1 large minced garlic clove. Keep chilled.

You might think of the lime on the glass rim as just a garnish. But, like nearly all garnishes, it should be eaten. So squirt that lime onto your cocktail. Don't just set it aside or eat around it.

FOOD FLAIR

For fruit fans, add more fresh lime juice and 1/2 cup diced fresh mango. For salad lovers, serve on a bed of mixed baby greens or mesclun. For garlic aficionados, use another garlic clove in the cocktail sauce.

FAST FIX

Prepare the Baja Shrimp Cocktail Sauce up to 2 days in advance. Store refrigerated in a covered container. Also, purchase precooked shrimp—fresh or frozen.

CARAMELIZED ANJOU PEAR, SAGE, AND GORGONZOLA QUESADILLA

Serves 4/serving size: 2 wedges

This is not your ooey, gooey, cheesy, fast-food quesadilla. It's a delicate appetizer. The fragrant sage will surely win you over. And the drizzling of honey is the ideal finishing touch.

- 1 large Anjou pear, cored, with skin, and very thinly sliced
- 4 (8-inch) whole wheat or regular flour tortillas
- 3 Tbsp finely crumbled gorgonzola cheese
- 8 large fresh sage leaves, thinly sliced (1 Tbsp)
- 2 tsp acacia or other mild floral honey

DIRECTIONS

1. Preheat the broiler. Arrange a single layer of pears on a large non-stick baking sheet. Lightly coat the pears with natural butter-flavored cooking spray. Broil for 2 to 3 minutes or until the pears begin to brown.

2. Lay the tortillas on a large baking sheet. Lightly coat with natural butter-flavored cooking spray. Turn two of the tortillas over. Divide the cheese, sage, and caramelized pears evenly over the entire surface of the turned-over tortillas. Top with remaining tortillas, sprayed sides up. Firmly press each quesadilla with your palm or a spatula to compact the ingredients.

3. Broil the quesadillas for 30 seconds or until toasted on top. Turn them over with a spatula and broil for another 30 seconds or until toasted on top. Watch them closely so they don't burn. (Alternatively, heat a large nonstick skillet over medium-high heat. Cook quesadillas one at a time for 2 minutes per side or until toasted.)

4. Cut each quesadilla into 4 wedges. Lightly drizzle with honey and serve warm.

Exchanges: 2 starch, 1/2 fruit, 1/2 fat; 170 calories, 20 calories from fat, 2 g total fat, 1 g saturated fat, 5 mg cholesterol, 320 mg sodium, 41 g total carbohydrate, 5 g dietary fiber, 9 g sugars, 6 g protein.

FRESH FACT

Most pear varieties can be found in the United States in only the fall and winter. Anjou pears are available during the spring, too. So, you can enjoy this French crepe-like quesadilla most of the year.

FOOD FLAIR

To kick up the flavor further, sprinkle the caramelized pears generously with freshly ground black pepper before topping with tortillas.

FRESH BABY SPINACH AND FETA QUESADILLA

Serves 6/serving size: 2 wedges

It looks Mexican—but it tastes Greek. And the unique combination makes these quesadillas burst with international flavor. Oopah! Olé!

- 1/2 cup packed fresh basil leaves
- 1 1/2 Tbsp lemon juice
- 1 Tbsp pine nuts
- 1 tsp extra virgin olive oil
- 1/4 tsp sea salt, or to taste
- 1/4 tsp freshly ground black pepper, or to taste
- 6 (8-inch) whole wheat or regular flour tortillas
- 1/3 cup finely crumbled natural feta cheese
- 1 cup finely chopped fresh organic baby spinach
- 3 Tbsp minced green onion (green part only)

DIRECTIONS

1. Place the basil, lemon juice, pine nuts, oil, salt, and pepper into a food processor and pulse until the mixture has a pesto-like consistency.

2. Lay the tortillas on a large baking sheet and lightly coat with natural butter-flavored cooking spray. Turn three of the tortillas over. Spread basil "pesto" over the entire surface of these tortillas. Sprinkle with cheese, spinach, and green onion. Top with the remaining tortillas, sprayed side up. Firmly press each quesadilla with your palm or a spatula to compact the ingredients.

3. Heat a large nonstick skillet over medium-high heat. Cook quesadillas in batches, 2 minutes per side, or until toasted. Cut each quesadilla into 4 wedges and serve warm.

Exchanges: 1 1/2 starch, 1 vegetable, 1/2 fat; 150 calories, 35 calories
from fat, 4 g total fat, 1 g saturated fat, 5 mg cholesterol, 430 mg sodium,
31 g total carbohydrate, 3 g dietary fiber, 1 g sugars, 6 g protein.

FRESH FACT

Feta cheese, the classic Greek curd cheese, has been enjoyed
for centuries. It's traditionally made with goat's or sheep's milk and
cured in brine. Cow's milk varieties are available, too—but they're
technically no longer true feta. Whichever you use, it'll add tanginess to
traditional and nontraditional cuisine alike. And because it's so flavorful, you don't need much to make any dish feta-licious.

CAPRESE PIZZETTE

Serves 6/serving size: 1 piece

Nutritious pizza? Yes, this one is! It's a fun food for parties. It's also ideal as a luscious bite alongside a satisfying salad for a light lunch. Kids will love it as an after-school snack, too.

- 2 (2-oz) whole wheat lavash flatbreads
- 2/3 cup lightly packed shredded part-skim mozzarella cheese
- 1 large beefsteak tomato, thinly sliced (about 8 slices)
- 1/4 tsp garlic salt, or to taste
- 1 Tbsp extra virgin olive oil
- 1/3 cup thinly sliced fresh basil leaves

DIRECTIONS

1. Preheat the broiler. Place the flatbreads on a large baking sheet and broil for 1 minute on each side or until lightly toasted. Remove from the oven and reduce the heat to 450°F.

2. Top the entire surface of each flatbread with cheese. Arrange tomatoes on top of the cheese and sprinkle with garlic salt. When the oven is ready, bake on the middle rack for 5 minutes or until the tomatoes are cooked through and the flatbreads are fully crisped.

3. Immediately drizzle with olive oil and sprinkle with basil. Cut each pizzette in half and serve immediately.

Exchanges: 1/2 starch, 1 vegetable, 1 fat; 100 calories, 40 calories from fat, 4 g total fat, 1 g saturated fat, 5 mg cholesterol, 200 mg sodium, 13 g total carbohydrate, 2 g dietary fiber, 1 g sugars, 5 g protein.

FOOD FLAIR

For extra pizzazz, lightly drizzle the tomatoes with aged balsamic vinegar at serving time.

ASIAN-STYLE PORK MEATBALLS

Serves 10/serving size: 2 meatballs

These meatballs are so good that you'll be surprised at how few calories they have . . . just 35 each! It's the soy sauce that provides the deliciousness called "umami." Now that's worth celebrating—and these perky meatballs are definitely party-worthy. Serve them with Zesty Orange–Ginger Dip (see recipe, page 64) for a yin-yang flavor appeal.

- 1 lb lean ground pork (antibiotic free)
- 2 Tbsp cold water
- 1/3 cup thinly sliced green onion
- 2 Tbsp whole wheat bread crumbs
- 2 Tbsp naturally brewed reduced-sodium soy sauce
- 1 large garlic clove, minced

DIRECTIONS

1. Preheat the oven to 425°F.

2. In a medium bowl, add all ingredients and combine with your hands, then make 20 meatballs (about 2 Tbsp mixture each). Moisten hands with water when forming the meatballs if the mixture becomes sticky.

3. Place the meatballs on a nonstick baking pan and bake 15 minutes or until done. Serve on toothpicks.

Exchanges: 1 lean meat, 1/2 fat; 70 calories, 23 calories from fat, 3 g total fat, 1 g saturated fat, 25 mg cholesterol, 140 mg sodium, 1 g total carbohydrate, 0 g dietary fiber, 0 g sugars, 10 g protein.

FOOD FLAIR

In a spicy mood? Add about 1/4 tsp each freshly ground black pepper and ground cayenne red pepper into the pork mixture before forming the meatballs.

PARTY PEANUT CHICKEN SATAY

Serves 8/serving size: 1 satay

*Anything that comes on a stick seems to taste better.
That might have something to do with the fun factor.
But skewer or no skewer, these party satays are peanutty good—
with just the right bite of spice.*

- 3 Tbsp naturally brewed reduced-sodium soy sauce
- 2 Tbsp organic coconut milk
- 1 1/2 Tbsp acacia or other mild floral honey
- 1 Tbsp Thai red curry paste

- 1 Tbsp rice vinegar
- 1 Tbsp water
- 1 tsp grated fresh ginger root
- 2 large garlic cloves, halved
- 15 fresh cilantro stems with leaves attached (do not chop)

- 1 lb unseasoned, uncooked chicken breast tenders or boneless, skinless chicken breast (antibiotic free), sliced lengthwise into 16 thin strips
- 2 Tbsp finely chopped salted, roasted peanuts

DIRECTIONS

1. In a small saucepan, stir together the soy sauce, coconut milk, honey, curry paste, vinegar, water, and ginger. Stir in the garlic and cilantro and bring to a boil over medium-high heat. Reduce heat to low and simmer for 5 minutes. Remove from heat and cool completely in the refrigerator.

MORE THAN FOUR?

If you want to serve these satays for a party, this recipe can feed 16—1 piece of chicken per 6-inch skewer instead of 2 pieces of chicken per larger skewer.

2. Place the chicken strips into a bowl or large plastic freezer bag, add the cold marinade, cover or seal, and marinate in the refrigerator for 2 or more hours, tossing after 1 hour to recoat. Meanwhile, soak 8 (10- or 12-inch) bamboo skewers in water for at least 30 minutes.

3. Preheat the oven to 350°F. Secure two chicken strips onto each skewer in a ribbon-like manner. Position the satays on a large nonstick baking pan. Sprinkle peanuts on top of the chicken. (Or, place the peanuts on a plate or tray and press the satays onto the peanuts. Place the satays on the pan peanut-coated side up.)

FRESH FACT

It's okay to marinate these chicken skewers overnight. They'll be a bit more tender and a little spicier. If you like your chicken mild, not wild, cut the red curry paste in half when making the marinade.

4. Roast on the middle oven rack for 20 minutes or until done. Serve warm. Garnish with additional fresh cilantro, if desired.

Exchanges: 1/2 carbohydrate, 2 lean meat; 110 calories, 31 calories from fat, 3 g total fat, 1 g saturated fat, 35 mg cholesterol, 310 mg sodium, 5 g total carbohydrate, 0 g dietary fiber, 3 g sugars, 14 g protein.

FOOD FLAIR

Make an Asian chicken salad. After the skewers are cooked, let them sit for 5 minutes. Remove the chicken from the skewers. Serve the chicken, warm or cold, on top of salad greens and drizzle with dressing, such as an Asian sesame, sesame–ginger, or cilantro–lime vinaigrette.

FOOD FLAIR

To please everyone's palate, use different nuts or seeds instead of sticking with peanuts. Try cashews or hazelnuts next time for a change of taste. Go organic with nuts if you choose, too. Organic cashews and other nuts are more widely available than ever before.

CHILI–LIME CRISPED CHICKEN FINGERS

Serves 4/serving size: 2 chicken fingers

These fun-to-eat "fingers" are tender, crispy, and extra spicy. With all of that flavor, you'll never miss the fat. Now that's hot!

- 1 Tbsp Asian garlic-chili sauce or other spicy Asian chili sauce
- 1 Tbsp lime juice
- 1 Tbsp clover honey
- 1/4 tsp sea salt, or to taste
- 1/4 tsp freshly ground black pepper, or to taste
- 10 oz unseasoned, uncooked chicken breast tenders or boneless, skinless chicken breast (antibiotic free), sliced into 8 wide, long strips
- 1/2 cup plain whole wheat panko bread crumbs

DIRECTIONS

1. Preheat the oven to 375°F. In a medium bowl, stir together the chili sauce, lime juice, honey, salt, and pepper. Add the chicken and toss until well coated.

2. Place the bread crumbs in a shallow bowl. One at a time, dip all sides of the chicken strips into the bread crumbs and place on a large nonstick baking pan.

3. Lightly coat the chicken strips with natural butter-flavored cooking spray, if desired. Bake for 22 minutes or until done. Let the chicken cool on the pan for 5 minutes before serving.

Exchanges: 1/2 carbohydrate, 2 lean meat; 130 calories, 17 calories from fat, 2 g total fat, 0 g saturated fat, 40 mg cholesterol, 190 mg sodium, 11 g total carbohydrate, 1 g dietary fiber, 4 g sugars, 16 g protein.

FRESH FACT

A nationwide survey conducted in 2005 found that American consumers eat chicken an average of five times in a two-week period. And chicken strips are one of the most popular ways to enjoy it.

FRESH FACT

Panko bread crumbs are traditionally used as a coating in fried Japanese cuisine. Since they're extra coarse, you'll especially like how they make these chicken fingers extra crispy.

CURRY CHICKEN BREAST SALAD WITH RED GRAPES IN WONTON CUPS

Serves 4/serving size: 3 wonton cups

Enjoy exotic-tasting chicken salad as a fun finger food. These fancy little cups will be a big hit at your next party.

- 12 wonton wrappers
- 1 cup finely diced, cooked boneless, skinless chicken breast (antibiotic free), chilled
- 1/4 cup plain fat-free yogurt
- 1 Tbsp mayonnaise
- 1 Tbsp mango chutney
- 1 tsp hot Madras curry powder
- 1/4 tsp sea salt, or to taste
- 3 Tbsp diced celery
- 1/2 cup seedless red grapes, thinly sliced horizontally
- 2 tsp minced fresh cilantro

DIRECTIONS

1. Preheat the oven to 350°F. Coat a nonstick mini-muffin tin with natural butter-flavored cooking spray and press a wonton square into each cup of the tin, forming a wonton cup. Lightly coat the wonton cups with cooking spray and bake for 12 minutes or until golden brown. Remove from the oven and let cool in the pan.

2. Meanwhile, in a medium bowl, stir together the chicken, yogurt, mayonnaise, chutney, curry powder, and salt. Then add the celery, grapes, and cilantro and stir.

3. With a spoon, stuff about 2 Tbsp of the salad into each wonton cup. Garnish each with a tiny sprig of cilantro or a red grape sliver, if desired.

Exchanges: 1 1/2 carbohydrate, 1 lean meat, 1/2 fat; 190 calories, 54 calories from fat, 6 g total fat, 1 g saturated fat, 35 mg cholesterol, 330 mg sodium, 20 g total carbohydrate, 1 g dietary fiber, 6 g sugars, 14 g protein.

FRESH FACTS

If you're preparing chicken just for this dish, poach or roast about 7 1/2 oz raw boneless, skinless chicken breast to yield 5 oz cooked. For a change of taste, try unsweetened tea as a unique poaching liquid.

FAST FIX

Use leftover chicken for this dish and it'll go speedy quick. Also, if you're using chicken that's already seasoned, then leave the salt out of this recipe.

FRESH FACTS

If you don't have or can't find mango chutney, replace it in this recipe with 1 Tbsp mango or apricot jam plus 1/2 tsp grated fresh ginger root.

MORE THAN FOUR?

Prepare this appetizer for a party. First, plan on your guests eating 1 or 2 filled wonton cups each, not 3. That's because you'll likely be serving other appetizers, too. Double or triple the recipe accordingly. Make the wonton cups and chicken salad up to 2 days in advance. Store unfilled wonton cups at room temperature in a tightly sealed container; store chicken salad refrigerated in a tightly sealed container. Fill the cups just before serving so the wontons stay crisp.

DAINTY TEA SANDWICHES

Serves 8/serving size: 2 sandwiches

There's no tea in these sandwiches, of course. But they're perfect bites to serve at teatime—along with your favorite hot or iced tea. The ladies will love these. Kids, too. Men can partake in this tasty pleasure, but it's probably best not to call the sandwiches "dainty" in their presence.

- 1/2 (12-inch) English (hot-house) cucumber with skin, thinly sliced
- 1/2 tsp sea salt
- 4 (1-oz) slices firm-textured whole wheat bread

- 4 (1-oz) slices firm-textured white or whole wheat bread
- 1 Tbsp unsalted butter, softened
- 2 tsp finely chopped fresh dill
- 1/4 tsp freshly ground black pepper, or to taste

- 2 Tbsp organic low-fat sour cream or plain fat-free Greek yogurt (or yogurt cheese; see recipe, page 63)
- 1/3 cup finely minced green onion (green part only)

DIRECTIONS

1. Arrange the cucumber slices in a single layer on a large plate. Sprinkle with salt. Cover the cucumber slices with another plate. Top the plate with weight, such as jars of condiments. Let stand for at least 2 hours in the refrigerator.

2. Drain the juices from the cucumber slices. Pat dry between layers of plain paper towels and refrigerate until ready to use.

3. Trim crusts from the bread slices. Lightly spread one side of each bread slice with butter. Top buttered side of 4 slices (2 whole wheat and 2 white, if using both types of bread) with cucumber slices, dill, and pepper to taste. Cover with remaining bread slices, buttered side down. Cut each sandwich diagonally into quarters.

4. With a butter knife, lightly spread sour cream or yogurt on one cut side of each sandwich quarter. Gently dip that side into the green onion.

Exchanges: 1 carbohydrate, 1/2 fat; 80 calories, 22 calories from fat, 2 g total fat, 1 g saturated fat, 5 mg cholesterol, 280 mg sodium, 11 g total carbohydrate, 1 g dietary fiber, 2 g sugars, 2 g protein.

FRESH FACT

Save the leftover bread crusts, chop or cube, and bake at 375°F for 15 minutes until crisp. Use as salad or stuffing croutons.

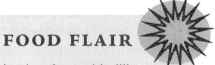

FOOD FLAIR

For a burst of fresh taste, add fresh mint along with dill.
For less daintiness, add a pinch of ground red cayenne pepper and garlic powder to the cucumbers along with the black pepper.

HAWAIIAN-STYLE EDAMAME

Serves 4/serving size: 1/4 recipe

Pure, simple, edible enjoyment. No lei, Hawaiian shirt, or grass skirt required.

- 1 (10-oz) bag frozen edamame (soybeans in the pod)
- 1/2 tsp coarse red Hawaiian or other coarse sea salt, or to taste

DIRECTIONS

1. Place a large saucepan filled about 3/4 full of water over high heat and bring to a boil. Add the frozen edamame and return to a boil, then boil for 3 minutes.

2. Remove the edamame with a slotted spoon to a bowl of ice water to stop the cooking process. Drain once the edamame is slightly cool. Trim each pod's stem end for easy eating.

3. While the edamame are still slightly moist, and just before serving, toss with salt. Provide bowls for the empty pods.

Exchanges: 1/2 starch, 1 lean meat; 90 calories, 26 calories from fat, 3 g total fat, 0 g saturated fat, 0 mg cholesterol, 320 mg sodium, 9 g total carbohydrate, 4 g dietary fiber, 1 g sugars, 8 g protein.

FRESH FACT

Edamame are fresh Japanese soybeans in their green pods. They're at their freshest best in the summer, but are easily found frozen year-round.

FOOD FLAIR

Experiment with different sea salts. Try Celtic gray sea salt, Italian sea salt, or fleur de sel. Each has a unique flavor. What's more, by finding a salt you love, you may be satisfied with less of it.

FAST FIX

You can prepare edamame up to 4 hours in advance. Keep them refrigerated in a bowl covered with a damp paper towel.

KOREAN FILET MIGNON "LOLLIPOPS"

Serves 8/serving size: 1 skewer

These savory, yet intriguingly sweet skewers are a healthier version of traditional Korean short ribs, called Kal Bi. In Korea, they'll be grilled. Since this recipe uses the tender and lean tenderloin, broiling works well, too. In fact, these brilliant beef "lollipops" are so tantalizing you'll want to make them again and again.

- 2 Tbsp naturally brewed reduced-sodium soy sauce
- 2 Tbsp packed organic brown sugar
- 3 Tbsp thinly sliced green onion
- 1 large garlic clove, minced
- 1 1/2 tsp grated fresh ginger root
- 1 tsp toasted sesame oil
- 1/4 tsp ground black pepper, or to taste
- 1 lb lean beef tenderloin (antibiotic free), trimmed of fat, sliced into 16 (1-oz) strips

DIRECTIONS

1. In a large bowl, stir together the soy sauce, brown sugar, green onion, garlic, ginger, oil, and pepper until well combined.

2. Place the beef strips into a bowl or large plastic freezer bag, add the marinade, cover or seal, and marinate in the refrigerator for 2 or more hours, tossing after 1 hour to recoat. Meanwhile, soak 8 (10- or 12-inch) bamboo skewers in water for at least 30 minutes.

3. Preheat the broiler or grill. Secure 2 beef strips onto each skewer. Drizzle meat with all remaining marinade. Cover the exposed ends of the skewers with foil. Broil or grill 2 to 3 minutes per side or until done as desired. Serve hot.

Exchanges: 2 lean meat; 100 calories, 32 calories from fat, 4 g total fat, 1 g saturated fat, 35 mg cholesterol, 180 mg sodium, 4 g total carbohydrate, 0 g dietary fiber, 3 g sugars, 12 g protein.

FRESH FACT

Ginger root is also just called ginger. We're much more familiar with the ground version, but for an unbelievable flavor boost, purchase fresh ginger that's firm and has smooth "skin." Before using, peel the "skin" with a vegetable peeler or the edge of a regular spoon. Then grate it using a Microplane® or box grater.

FOOD FLAIR

Immediately after grilling or broiling, sprinkle beef skewers with toasted or roasted sesame seeds. This adds eye appeal, a little crunch, and brings out full sesame flavor.

FAST FIX

Since they have such flavorful ingredients, these skewers are almost as enjoyable when you marinate them for 2 minutes instead of 2 hours. Just toss the beef with the marinade, skewer, and cook immediately.

MORE THAN FOUR?

If you want to serve these for a big party, this recipe can feed 16—1 strip of beef on each skewer. Also, consider cooking the beef without skewers, then simply insert a popsicle stick into each strip. It makes for a fun presentation—kid-friendly, too.

MINTED MIDDLE EASTERN MEATBALLS

Serves 4/serving size: 3 meatballs

A popular Lebanese dish is called kibbeh. Here, it's turned into a fabulous finger food using bread crumbs instead of bulgur wheat, plus tomato juice and yogurt to make it super moist. It's hard not to love these meatballs. They're natural party stars—especially when served with yogurt or dip.

- 10 oz extra lean ground beef or lean ground lamb (antibiotic free)
- 1/2 cup plain whole wheat bread crumbs
- 1/2 cup grated red or white onion
- 1/4 cup finely chopped fresh mint
- 2 Tbsp tomato or vegetable juice
- 2 Tbsp plain fat-free yogurt
- 1 tsp extra virgin olive oil
- 1/2 tsp sea salt
- 1/2 tsp ground cinnamon
- 1/4 tsp ground cumin

DIRECTIONS

1. Preheat the oven to 500°F. In a large bowl, add all ingredients and combine with your hands; then make 12 meatballs (about 3 Tbsp mixture each).

2. Place the meatballs on a medium nonstick baking pan and bake for 12 minutes or until cooked through.

3. Serve warm on toothpicks. Or serve on top of Greek yogurt (or yogurt cheese; see recipe, page 63) or Minted English Cucumber Tzatziki Dip (see recipe, page 62).

Exchanges: 1 carbohydrate, 2 lean meat; 170 calories, 44 calories from fat, 5 g total fat, 1 g saturated fat, 35 mg cholesterol, 360 mg sodium, 14 g total carbohydrate, 2 g dietary fiber, 2 g sugars, 18 g protein

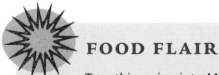

FRESH FACT

When finely chopping fresh mint or other herbs, make sure the leaves are dry for easier chopping. Use a sharp chef's knife, too.

FOOD FLAIR

Insert a few pan-toasted pine nuts into the middle of each meatball when forming the mixture into balls. It's kind of like a nutty surprise inside!

FOOD FLAIR

Turn this recipe into Middle Eastern Burgers. Grill or sauté the patties and serve in pita bread—or as is. Minted English Cucumber Tzatziki Dip (see recipe, page 62) makes a tasty condiment for the burgers, too.

ROASTED BEET AND ARTISANAL BLUE CHEESE SALSA IN ENDIVE

Serves 4/serving size: 3 stuffed endive leaves

This appetizer may be the tastiest way you've ever had beets. And it's so pretty.

- 1 tsp aged red wine vinegar
- 1 tsp extra virgin olive oil
- 2 Tbsp finely crumbled Artisanal blue cheese

- 3 medium beets, roasted, peeled, chilled, and cut into 1/8-inch cubes (about 1 1/2 cups; see Fresh Fact)
- 3 Tbsp golden raisins, minced

- 1 Tbsp minced green onion (white part only)
- 1/4 tsp sea salt, or to taste
- 1/8 tsp freshly ground black pepper, or to taste

- 1 head Belgian endive
- 3 Tbsp minced green onion (green part only)
- 2 tsp finely chopped, pan-toasted walnuts

DIRECTIONS

1. In a medium bowl, gently stir together the vinegar, oil, cheese, beets, raisins, white part of the green onion, salt, and pepper.

2. Cut the bottom from the endive, separate the leaves, rinse, and pat dry. Select the 12 nicest leaves.

3. Just before serving, place about 2 Tbsp of the beet–blue cheese salsa onto each leaf. Sprinkle with green onion and walnuts.

Exchanges: 1 carbohydrate, 1/2 fat; 100 calories, 30 calories from fat, 3 g total fat, 1 g saturated fat, 5 mg cholesterol, 260 mg sodium, 17 g total carbohydrate, 3 g dietary fiber, 11 g sugars, 3 g protein.

FRESH FACT

Artisanal cheese is made in small batches based on
time-honored traditions, recipes, and techniques.
American-made Artisanal blue cheeses include Great Hill Blue,
Bayley Hazen Blue, and Crater Lake Blue.

FRESH FACT

You can usually use organic canned beets
to save time. However, this recipe is best with
freshly roasted beets. To roast, preheat the oven
to 375°F. Cut green stems off beets, leaving
about 1/2 inch of the stem end on. Wrap each
beet in aluminum foil. Bake for 1 hour or until
done. Carefully remove foil to let the steam out.
Once beets are cool enough to handle, cut off
stems, sit beats on flat stem ends, and scrape
off peel with the back edge of a paring knife.
Then cube. You may want to wear gloves, since
beet juice stains. Store beets in a covered
container in the refrigerator for up to 2 days.

STUFFED BAKED POTATO SKINS WITH TURKEY BACON

Serves 4/serving size: 1 stuffed potato half

Potato skins are a restaurant classic, but often highly caloric. This rustic version is friendlier for the meal plan and zestier for the palate.

- 2 medium russet potatoes, baked and cooled (see Fresh Fact)
- 1/2 tsp garlic salt (divided use)
- 2 Tbsp shredded extra sharp or sharp cheddar cheese
- 1/2 cup thinly sliced green onion
- 2 Tbsp organic low-fat sour cream
- 1 (1-oz) slice organic turkey bacon, cooked crisp according to package directions, chopped into bits
- 1/8 tsp ground cayenne red pepper, or to taste

DIRECTIONS

1. Preheat the oven to 450°F. Cut each baked, cooled potato lengthwise into halves. Scoop out the centers and place in a medium bowl, leaving a 1/2-inch-thick potato layer on the skins. Place potato skins, cut sides up, on a nonstick baking sheet and sprinkle with 1/4 tsp garlic salt.

2. Add the remaining ingredients to the medium bowl and stir with a spoon until lightly mashed. Lightly pack the potato–cheese mixture on top of the potato skins.

3. Bake for 12 minutes or until the skins are crisp and the potato–cheese mixture is hot and begins to brown. Transfer potato skins to a platter and serve hot.

Exchanges: 1 1/2 starch; 120 calories, 22 calories from fat, 2 g total fat, 1 g saturated fat, 10 mg cholesterol, 190 mg sodium, 21 g total carbohydrate, 2 g dietary fiber, 2 g sugars, 4 g protein.

FRESH FACT

To bake potatoes, preheat the oven to 425°F. Scrub potatoes and pat dry. Pierce skins a few times each with a fork. Place potatoes on baking sheet and bake 45 minutes or until tender.

FAST FIX

Bake the potatoes up to 2 days in advance and store in the refrigerator.

MINI BURGERS WITH CARAMELIZED ONION

Serves 6/serving size: 1 burger

The caramelized onions give big-sized taste to these baby-sized burgers. Plus, they provide so much moistness and pleasant sweetness, you'll forget this savory, mini-meat cuisine is lean.

- 2 tsp canola oil
- 3 cups thinly sliced Vidalia, Maui, or other sweet onion
- 1/2 tsp sea salt, or to taste (divided use)
- 12 oz lean ground beef sirloin (antibiotic free)
- 1 Tbsp organic ketchup
- 1 1/2 tsp steak sauce
- 1 large garlic clove, minced
- 1/4 tsp freshly ground black pepper, or to taste
- 6 (1 1/2-oz) soft whole grain or other soft dinner rolls
- 6–12 organic baby arugula leaves, or to taste (optional)

DIRECTIONS

1. Preheat the broiler or grill. Heat the oil in a large nonstick skillet over medium heat. Add the onion and 1/4 tsp salt. Cook, stirring constantly, for 15 minutes or until golden brown.

2. In a medium bowl, add the beef, ketchup, steak sauce, garlic, 1/4 tsp salt, and pepper and combine with your hands until just mixed. Form into 6 burgers.

3. Broil or grill 1 minute per side or until medium well. (Remember, these burgers are lean and little, so they can dry out quickly with overcooking.) Remove from heat and let the burgers sit for 3 to 5 minutes before placing in buns. Top each beef patty with about 2 Tbsp caramelized onion and 1 to 2 arugula leaves (if using). Serve with additional organic ketchup or other condiment of choice.

Exchanges: 1 1/2 starch, 1 vegetable, 1 lean meat, 1/2 fat; 210 calories, 52 calories from fat, 6 g total fat, 1 g saturated fat, 20 mg cholesterol, 450 mg sodium, 24 g total carbohydrate, 4 g dietary fiber, 5 g sugars, 15 g protein.

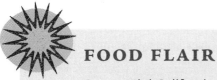

FOOD FLAIR

Create Mini California-Style Burgers with Caramelized Onion. Just before serving, slice up some Hass avocado, add a pinch of sea salt, and place in burgers. You won't need ketchup or other condiments.

FAST FIX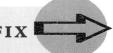

Prepare caramelized onions a day in advance. Store refrigerated in a covered bowl. Let them sit at room temperature 30 minutes before serving on the burgers.

LEMONY STUFFED GRAPE LEAVES

Serves 10/serving size: 2 large or 3 medium stuffed leaves

Lebanese cuisine is a traditionally fresh, flavorful, and natural cuisine that celebrates the goodness of life. Lebanese meals typically start with a mezze, which might include stuffed grape leaves (with or without meat), tabbouleh and other salads, hummus, kibbeh (a lamb dish), pita bread, and more. All together, these appetizers can make a balanced and beautiful meal.

- 1 1/4 cups brown basmati rice
- 3 large shallots, minced (1/2 cup)
- 1/4 cup finely chopped fresh dill
- 1/4 cup finely chopped fresh mint

- 1 1/2 tsp sea salt
- 3/4 tsp freshly ground black pepper, or to taste
- 1/4 cup water
- 3 medium lemons

- 30 medium or 20 large fresh grape leaves, lightly blanched (see Fresh Fact), or 1 (15-oz) jar grape leaves in vinegar brine, soaked in fresh water, rinsed well, and drained
- 1 Tbsp extra virgin olive oil

DIRECTIONS

1. In a medium mixing bowl, combine the rice, shallots, dill, mint, salt, and pepper. Add the water and stir to combine. Squeeze the juice from 1 1/2 lemons (to yield 5 Tbsp juice) into a small bowl and set aside. Cut the remaining lemons into small wedges.

2. Lay the grape leaves individually, dull side up, onto plain paper towels. If any leaves have stems attached, snip with thumbnail or kitchen shears. Place 1 heaping spoonful of the rice mixture in the center of each leaf. Roll each leaf tightly by folding the bottom end of each leaf over the filling, folding the edges over the filling, then rolling toward the leaf point, until they look like mini cigars.

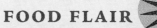

Wrap vegetables, meat, fish, or cheese with fresh grape leaves, then grill. Fresh leaves make a beautiful natural garnish for fruit and cheese platters, too.

3. In a large, heavy-duty saucepan, arrange the stuffed leaves in layers. (If you don't have a heavy-duty pan, line the pan's bottom with several large, unstuffed grape leaves before arranging the stuffed leaves on top.) Pour water (about 3 cups) over the rolls until just covered. Pour the lemon juice and oil evenly over all.

4. Place a heavy, heatproof plate or smaller pan lid directly onto the grape leaves to keep them from opening up during cooking. Place over high heat and bring to a boil. Cover the saucepan with a lid, reduce heat to low, and cook for 1 hour and 15 minutes, or until the rice is tender. Remove from heat and keep covered for 15 minutes. Serve warm or at room temperature with lemon wedges. They are delicious with plain Greek yogurt.

Exchanges: 1 starch, 1 vegetable, 1/2 fat; 110 calories, 21 calories from fat, 2 g total fat, 0 g saturated fat, 0 mg cholesterol, 350 mg sodium, 21 g total carbohydrate, 2 g dietary fiber, 1 g sugars, 3 g protein.

FRESH FACTS

To store grape leaves, stack 30 fresh leaves (make sure they're dry) and wrap the stack in plain paper towels. Then wrap in foil and place in a sealed plastic freezer bag. They'll keep frozen for months. When ready to use, remove from freezer and allow leaves to completely thaw. Rinse well with warm water to clean and lightly blanch the grape leaves.

Depending on where you live, fresh grape leaves are typically best picked from vines in the spring. (I'm half Lebanese, and grew up with grape vines in my backyard—for the leaves, not the grapes!) They'll likely be too tough by July 4. Select young whole leaves from wild or domesticated vines. Wild leaves are often more delicate and will result in a nicer finished dish.

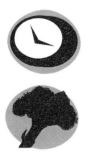

WHITE BEAN 'N' ROSEMARY BRUSCHETTA BITES

Serves 8/serving size: 3 bruschetta bites

Beans don't have a sexy image. That'll change after you experience these bites with their velvety topping. Oh, baby!

- 1 (15-oz) can organic cannellini or Great Northern beans, well drained
- 1 large garlic clove
- 2 Tbsp lemon juice, or to taste

- 1 Tbsp extra virgin olive oil
- 1/2 tsp finely chopped fresh rosemary leaves
- 1/4 tsp sea salt, or to taste

- 1 (6-oz) French baguette, cut into 24 (1/2-inch-thick) slices, discarding bread ends
- 2 large garlic cloves, peeled and cut in half

DIRECTIONS

1. Preheat the broiler. Puree the beans, garlic, lemon juice, oil, rosemary, and salt in a blender until smooth. If necessary, add 1 to 2 Tbsp cold water until bean mixture is desired consistency. (Be patient with the blending process, scraping down sides as needed. The thicker the bean puree, the better.)

2. Taste the puree and add more lemon or salt, if needed, as the sodium content and flavor of bean types vary. Refrigerate until ready to serve. (This bean topping is tasty when served either cool or at room temperature.)

3. Broil the baguette slices 20 to 30 seconds per side or until toasted. Once toasted, immediately rub the bread pieces with the cut end of the garlic.

4. Just before serving, dollop (don't spread) puree on top of each toast. If desired, garnish the platter with rosemary sprigs or each bruschetta bite with a few rosemary leaves.

Exchanges: 1 1/2 starch; 120 calories, 19 calories from fat, 2 g total fat, 0 g saturated fat, 0 mg cholesterol, 270 mg sodium, 20 g total carbohydrate, 3 g dietary fiber, 1 g sugars, 5 g protein.

FRESH FACT

Generally, a baguette refers to a long skinny loaf of white French bread. This recipe can be prepared using other varieties of bread, including whole wheat or sourdough. However, the airy texture of white French bread seems to pair best with this light topping.

FAST FIX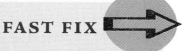

You can refrigerate the puree up to 3 days. (Refrigerating will help the puree to thicken slightly, too.) Toast the bread slices and store in a sealed plastic bag at room temperature up to 3 days. Make each serving at home as you need it. Or, to serve at a gathering, bring the puree and toasts packed separately. Prepare in a jiffy when you arrive at your destination.

CIABATTA BRUSCHETTA

Serves 16/serving size: 1 piece

If it's summer or fall, it's bruschetta time. The fresh tomatoes in it will be at their nutritional and flavorful best. And by using all high-quality, flavorful ingredients, you'll find you need less salt— or maybe no salt. That's amore for the heart.

- 1 (1-lb) loaf ciabatta bread or crusty Italian bread, cut into 16 slices
- 2 large garlic cloves, one cut in half, one minced
- 5 medium vine-ripened tomatoes, seeded and finely diced (2 1/2 cups)
- 1/3 cup thinly sliced green onion
- 3 Tbsp thinly sliced fresh basil leaves
- 1 Tbsp extra virgin olive oil
- 2 tsp aged red wine or balsamic vinegar
- 3/4 tsp sea salt, or to taste
- 1/2 tsp freshly ground pepper, or to taste

DIRECTIONS

1. Preheat the oven to 450°F. Toast bread slices on a nonstick baking sheet for 12 minutes or until lightly browned, turning bread over midway through toasting. Remove from the oven. While toast pieces are still warm, rub the top of each with the cut side of the garlic.

2. Meanwhile, stir the remaining ingredients together in a medium bowl. Allow to sit for at least 30 minutes. When ready to serve, stir, then place 2 1/2 Tbsp topping on each bread piece. Garnish platter with fresh basil or rosemary sprigs, if desired.

Exchanges: 1 starch; 90 calories, 18 calories from fat, 2 g total fat, 0 g saturated fat, 0 mg cholesterol, 280 mg sodium, 16 g total carbohydrate, 1 g dietary fiber, 2 g sugars, 3 g protein.

FRESH FACT

Ciabatta, which actually means "slipper," is a crusty Italian white bread. It's okay to eat small amounts of white bread on occasion—especially when it tastes better with the recipe or is a tradition. Simply remember to make at least half your daily grain choices from whole grains. Better yet, if you have a nearby Italian bakery, look for ciabatta integrale, the whole wheat version of this bread.

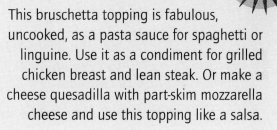

FOOD FLAIR

This bruschetta topping is fabulous, uncooked, as a pasta sauce for spaghetti or linguine. Use it as a condiment for grilled chicken breast and lean steak. Or make a cheese quesadilla with part-skim mozzarella cheese and use this topping like a salsa.

FAST FIX

Use organic canned diced tomatoes in the winter or spring in place of the fresh vine-ripened tomatoes.

GRILLED VEGETABLE PALETTE

Serves 4/serving size: 3 veggie pieces

At just 6% of the daily value for total fat, this veggie plate is totally phat! Adults will go crazy for their veggies this way. Kids might, too.

- 1/2 cup packed fresh basil leaves
- 2 large garlic cloves
- 2 Tbsp natural vegetable broth
- 1 Tbsp aged balsamic vinegar
- 1 Tbsp extra virgin olive oil (divided use)
- 1/2 tsp sea salt
- 1/4 tsp freshly ground black pepper, or to taste
- 1 large zucchini or yellow squash with skin, sliced lengthwise into 4 large strips
- 1 medium eggplant with skin, sliced lengthwise into 4 large strips
- 1 large red bell pepper, sliced lengthwise into 4 large strips

DIRECTIONS

1. Preheat the grill over medium-high heat. Puree the basil, garlic, broth, vinegar, 1 tsp oil, salt, and pepper in a blender for 1 minute or until smooth.

2. Place the vegetables in a large sealable plastic bag and add the basil puree. Seal and shake the bag until all vegetables are well coated. Grill vegetables 4 to 5 minutes per side or until lightly charred and cooked through, turning only as needed.

3. Arrange the vegetables onto a platter as if it's an artist's palette. Drizzle with remaining oil. Serve with additional balsamic vinegar on the side and garnish with fresh sliced basil, if desired. Serve at room temperature.

Exchanges: 2 vegetable, 1 fat; 80 calories, 35 calories from fat, 4 g total fat, 1 g saturated fat, 0 mg cholesterol, 310 mg sodium, 12 g total carbohydrate, 4 g dietary fiber, 6 g sugars, 2 g protein.

FRESH FACT

Think locally when choosing fresh; think globally when buying the rest. Go for the highest quality, most flavorful ingredients—they're often the most nutritious. Consider an extra virgin olive oil from Spain, the country where olive trees thrive and the source of most of the world's olive oil. Choose aged balsamic vinegar from the Modena or Reggio regions in Italy. If it's not from there, it's not "real" balsamic vinegar from 100% Trebbiano grapes— and it might have added brown sugar or other ingredients.

FAST FIX

Vegetables can be grilled (outdoors or in) up to 2 hours in advance. Let stand at room temperature. Refrigerate leftovers up to 2 days and savor in sandwiches, or chop and toss into pasta.

FOOD FLAIR

Instead of creating an artist's palette, layer all vegetables into two stacks when serving. For instance, from the bottom to the top of the stack, layer eggplant, red pepper, zucchini; repeat. For added interest, tuck fresh basil leaves between the layers.

FAST FIXES

Don't want to mess with the grill? Place a grill pan over medium-high heat. Once hot, add veggies in batches. Cook 4 minutes per side or until done as desired. Or in a panini-style indoor grill on medium-high heat, grill in three batches—cooking all like vegetables, such as all eggplant slices, together. That will assure even cooking, since the vegetables are of different thicknesses. Cook each batch 5-6 minutes total or until done as desired.

MEXICAN SPA "SPRING ROLLS"

Serves 15/serving size: 1 roll

These "spring rolls" are good-looking—and good-tasting. The delectable secret: combining a naturally lighter product (Neufchâtel cheese) with "heat" (jalapeño). Go for hot salsa, too … if you dare! Luckily this is a seemingly rich appetizer—or spatizer—to which you won't need to say "no." It's a crowd-pleaser at parties, too.

- 4 oz Neufchâtel cheese (light cream cheese)
- 3 Tbsp natural salsa (mild, medium, or hot), excess liquid drained
- 1 small jalapeño pepper with seeds, minced
- 1/4 cup minced green onion
- 2 Tbsp finely chopped fresh cilantro
- 5 (8-inch) whole wheat or regular flour tortillas
- 15 fresh cilantro leaves

DIRECTIONS

1. Using an electric mixer, thoroughly combine the cream cheese, salsa, jalapeño, green onion, and cilantro in a small mixing bowl.

2. With a small flexible spatula or butter knife, spread about 3 Tbsp filling over the entire surface of each tortilla. Roll each up tightly (see Fast Fix).

3. Slice about 1/2 inch off each end of the rolled tortillas. Then diagonally slice each rolled tortilla into 3 equal pieces.

4. Stand each sliced piece on a cut edge and garnish the top with a cilantro leaf. Cover with plastic wrap and refrigerate until ready to serve.

Exchanges: 1/2 starch; 45 calories, 17 calories from fat, 2 g total fat, 1 g saturated fat, 5 mg cholesterol, 105 mg sodium, 7 g total carbohydrate, 1 g dietary fiber, 1 g sugars, 2 g protein.

FRESH FACT

Don't worry about whether your salsa is made in Mexico, Memphis, or Manhattan. Rather, worry about the ingredients that go into it. Often, the best tasting salsa has the fewest ingredients. Make your own salsa if you prefer. Try Tomato-Cilantro Salsa Fresca (see recipe, page 71)—just drain, then puree it for best results in this recipe.

FOOD FLAIR

Serve these like sushi. Slice each filled and rolled tortilla into 6 pieces instead of 3. Serve 2 pieces of "sushi" per person, along with chopsticks. And, be sure to have 30 fresh cilantro leaves for topping each piece.

FAST FIX

For best results, after spreading the tortillas with the cream cheese mixture and rolling, wrap them in plastic wrap and refrigerate for at least 15 minutes; this allows for easier slicing. If you choose, this step can be done 1 day in advance.

TOSSED

BROCCOLI LAYER SALAD WITH DRIED CRANBERRIES

Serves 6/serving size: 1 1/2 cups

A more caloric version of this crunchy salad has been around for decades. You'll want this beautifully balanced, diabetes-friendly version around for decades more in your recipe repertoire. It's packed with nutrients, including antioxidants. In fact, each serving provides over 100% of your daily need for vitamin C. Move over, orange juice!

- 8 cups bite-size broccoli florets
- 1 cup thinly sliced red onion
- 1/3 cup dried cranberries
- 1/3 cup freshly shredded extra sharp or sharp cheddar cheese
- 1/2 cup plain fat-free yogurt
- 2 Tbsp apple cider vinegar
- 2 Tbsp acacia or other mild floral honey
- 1 Tbsp mayonnaise
- 2 Tbsp salted sunflower seeds, roasted or toasted

DIRECTIONS

1. In a large glass trifle or serving bowl, layer the broccoli, onion, cranberries, and cheese.

2. In a small bowl, whisk the yogurt, vinegar, honey, and mayonnaise. Pour the dressing evenly over the salad.

3. Cover and refrigerate. Sprinkle with sunflower seeds just before serving.

Exchanges: 1 carbohydrate, 1 fat; 130 calories, 49 calories from fat, 5 g total fat, 1 g saturated fat, 5 mg cholesterol, 95 mg sodium, 18 g total carbohydrate, 3 g dietary fiber, 11 g sugars, 5 g protein.

FOOD FLAIR

For added appeal, cook 3 (1-oz) slices organic turkey bacon until crisp, chop into bits, and sprinkle on top of the salad when ready to serve. For flavor variety, use chopped, toasted walnuts or dry-roasted peanuts. And if you have a favorite dried fruit other than cranberries, use it instead. Dried tart cherries or thinly sliced dried plums work wonderfully.

CREOLE FINGERLING POTATO SALAD

Serves 6/serving size: scant 1 cup

Creole is all about full flavor. And, when Creole mustard is added to the cute banana-shaped potatoes, it creates potato salad perfection. It's something to definitely get jazzed up about.

- 1 3/4 lb banana fingerling potatoes, unpeeled
- 3/4 cup thinly sliced celery (slice on diagonal)
- 3 Tbsp Creole or spicy Dijon mustard
- 2 Tbsp organic low-fat sour cream
- 2 Tbsp mayonnaise
- 1/4 cup chopped fresh chives (divided use)
- 1 Tbsp chopped fresh dill
- 1/4 tsp sea salt, or to taste

DIRECTIONS

1. Add the potatoes to a large saucepan or stockpot and cover with cold water. Bring to a boil and cook for 20 minutes or until just tender, making sure the potatoes are always submerged in water. Drain and let cool, then slice into 1/4-inch-thick rounds. Transfer to a large bowl and stir in the celery.

2. In a small bowl, combine the mustard, sour cream, mayonnaise, 3 Tbsp chives, and dill, then stir into the potato mixture. Stir in salt, then cover and chill at least 30 minutes to allow flavors to blend.

3. Sprinkle with remaining chives and serve.

Exchanges: 1 1/2 starch, 1/2 fat; 140 calories, 38 calories from fat, 4 g total fat, 1 g saturated fat, 5 mg cholesterol, 240 mg sodium, 23 g total carbohydrate, 3 g dietary fiber, 2 g sugars, 3 g protein.

FRESH FACT

If you're not on an eating plan that specifically restricts sodium, this tip's for you. If you keep your sodium intake low throughout the day, it's probably okay to boil these potatoes in salted water—it'll boost the potato flavor.

FAST FIX

You can make this salad 1 day ahead—just keep it refrigerated. It's actually better the next day, after all the flavors have married. If you plan to serve this in a day or two, stir the celery in just before serving for optimal crispness.

MORE THAN FOUR?

Double or triple this recipe to take it to a large picnic gathering or barbecue party. Just make sure you have a stockpot large enough to boil all the potatoes. And remember to keep the salad chilled until you're ready to serve. Perishable foods—those normally requiring refrigeration—should not sit outside for more than 2 hours or, if it's above 90°F outside, just 1 hour.

FRESH BABY SPINACH ORZO SALAD WITH GOAT CHEESE

Serves 4/serving size: 1 1/2 cups

It's okay to enjoy regular pasta, like orzo, on occasion—without guilt. Sometimes it simply tastes better than whole wheat pasta when paired with certain ingredients . . . as in this salad. It's important to maintain enjoyment in your meals. Just remember to eat mostly whole grains the rest of the day.

- 5 oz dry orzo (7/8 cup)
- 2 Tbsp lemon juice
- 1 Tbsp extra virgin olive oil
- 3/4 tsp sea salt, or to taste
- 2 cups fresh organic baby spinach
- 1/3 cup thinly sliced green onion
- 1 cup grape tomatoes, halved vertically
- 1/4 cup thinly sliced fresh basil leaves
- 3 Tbsp finely crumbled soft goat cheese
- 1 Tbsp pine nuts, pan-toasted

DIRECTIONS

1. Cook orzo according to package directions, omitting added oil and salt. Drain.

2. In a large bowl, whisk the lemon juice, oil, and salt. Add the hot orzo to the dressing and toss. Chill, stirring occasionally to help prevent sticking.

3. When the orzo is cool, add the spinach, green onion, tomatoes, and basil and toss. Sprinkle with goat cheese and pine nuts. Serve at room temperature or chilled.

Exchanges: 1 1/2 starch, 1 vegetable, 1 fat; 200 calories, 59 calories from fat, 7 g total fat, 1 g saturated fat, 0 mg cholesterol, 470 mg sodium, 31 g total carbohydrate, 3 g dietary fiber, 3 g sugars, 7 g protein.

FRESH FACT

A person with diabetes is at greater risk for developing heart disease. So eating foods rich in heart-protective nutrients is important. That's where spinach comes in. It's one of the best natural sources of folate, a nutrient that may reduce the risk of heart disease, as well as stroke and birth defects.

FOOD FLAIR

Instead of just basil, use a mixture of fresh herbs, such as flat-leaf parsley, mint, and basil. And instead of baby spinach, go for a peppery kick with organic baby arugula. It's good for you, too.

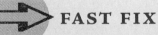

FAST FIX

Even if you're making this for one or two people, go ahead and make the full recipe. It keeps well, covered, in the refrigerator for a couple of days. Enjoy it as an entrée or side, with lunch or dinner, or just as a snack.

HEIRLOOM TOMATO SALAD

Serves 4/serving size: 1 salad (10 to 12 tomato slices)

Heirloom tomatoes are from open-pollinated heirloom seeds. Heirloom fruits and vegetables, including tomatoes, are known for their full-bodied flavors. The tomatoes are delicious simply eaten alone. Imagine how good they'll be complemented by the other fresh and fabulous ingredients in this salad.

- 4 large heirloom tomatoes of assorted colors, thinly sliced (10 to 12 slices each)
- 3/4 cup thinly sliced red onion
- 2 Tbsp aged balsamic vinegar
- 1 1/2 tsp extra virgin olive oil
- 1/2 tsp sea salt, or to taste
- 1/4 tsp freshly ground black pepper, or to taste
- 1/4 cup thinly sliced fresh basil leaves or 2 Tbsp minced fresh chives

DIRECTIONS

1. Arrange the tomatoes on a platter, overlapping and alternating colors. Scatter the onion on top of the tomatoes.

2. In a small bowl, whisk the vinegar and oil. Drizzle the dressing over the tomatoes and sprinkle with salt, pepper, and basil or chives.

Exchanges: 1 carbohydrate, 1/2 fat; 90 calories, 22 calories from fat, 2 g total fat, 0 g saturated fat, 0 mg cholesterol, 310 mg sodium, 16 g total carbohydrate, 4 g dietary fiber, 10 g sugars, 3 g protein.

FRESH FACT

Enjoy plenty of fresh tomato dishes in the summer when tomatoes are in season. To make sure tomatoes stay at their flavorful best, don't refrigerate them. Refrigerating tomatoes strips them of their flavor and makes them mealy.

FAST FIX

If you can't find heirloom tomatoes, buy vine-ripened or beefsteak tomatoes. Make sure they're completely ripe before making this salad.

FOOD FLAIR

Sprinkle each serving with 1 Tbsp finely crumbled soft goat cheese. Or, for a more extravagant presentation, lightly brush 8 (3/4-inch-thick) slices crusty bread with extra virgin olive oil. Grill the bread slices for 2 to 3 minutes per side, or until browned as desired. Immediately rub toasts with garlic halves and serve topped with Heirloom Tomato Salad. Garnish the platter with fresh basil leaves.

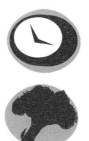

HIBACHI SLAW

Serves 4/serving size: 1 cup

Even the staunchest of coleslaw critics might be converted back to fans after a bite of this Asian-styled slaw. It's a memorable showcase of sweet and savory. And the honey-roasted nuts are a highlight.

- 3 cups shredded green cabbage
- 1 cup fresh mung bean sprouts
- 1/3 cup thinly sliced green onion (slice on diagonal)
- 2 Tbsp chopped fresh cilantro
- 3 Tbsp natural low-fat ginger-flavored or other Asian-style vinaigrette
- 1 Tbsp naturally brewed reduced-sodium soy sauce
- 1 Tbsp acacia or other mild floral honey
- 1/4 tsp freshly ground black pepper, or to taste
- 1/3 cup honey-roasted almonds or peanuts, chopped

DIRECTIONS

1. In a large bowl, combine the cabbage, bean sprouts, green onion, and cilantro.

2. In a small bowl, whisk the vinaigrette, soy sauce, honey, and pepper.

3. Add the vinaigrette mixture to the coleslaw and toss. Sprinkle with nuts and garnish with a fresh cilantro sprig, if desired. Serve immediately. Enjoy with chopsticks.

Exchanges: 1 carbohydrate, 1 fat; 130 calories, 61 calories from fat, 7 g total fat, 1 g saturated fat, 0 mg cholesterol, 280 mg sodium, 15 g total carbohydrate, 4 g dietary fiber, 8 g sugars, 5 g protein.

FRESH FACT

Speed eating can result in overeating. Here's a fix for fast eaters. Use chopsticks to slow down your eating rate—and not just with Asian food. Start the habit with this slaw. But if you get too skilled with your chopsticks, you might need to find another trick.

FOOD FLAIR

Garnish this slaw with crispy wonton strips, if desired. Slice 4 wonton wrappers into 10 thin strips each. Place the strips on a baking sheet and lightly coat with natural cooking spray. Bake in a 400°F oven for 5 minutes or until crisp and golden brown.

FAST FIX

Instead of buying, rinsing, and shredding cabbage, pick up an 8-oz package of coleslaw mix from the produce department.

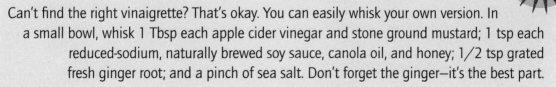

FOOD FLAIR

Can't find the right vinaigrette? That's okay. You can easily whisk your own version. In a small bowl, whisk 1 Tbsp each apple cider vinegar and stone ground mustard; 1 tsp each reduced-sodium, naturally brewed soy sauce, canola oil, and honey; 1/2 tsp grated fresh ginger root; and a pinch of sea salt. Don't forget the ginger—it's the best part.

JALAPEÑO SOY CAESAR SALAD WITH BLACKENED CHICKEN BREAST

Serves 4/serving size: 3 cups

If you want authentic Caesar salad, this entrée-sized recipe isn't it. But if you want something that's a little bit different, this might just knock your socks off! It can even knock the socks off most vegetarians—it's equally fabulous without the chicken.

- 1 lb boneless, skinless chicken breasts (antibiotic free)
- 1 1/2 tsp extra virgin olive oil (divided use)
- 1 tsp freshly ground black pepper, or to taste (divided use)
- 1 small jalapeño pepper with seeds
- 3 large garlic cloves
- 1/4 cup grated Parmigiana-Reggiano cheese
- 2 Tbsp Dijon mustard
- 1 1/2 Tbsp Worcestershire sauce
- 4 oz soft silken tofu, drained (1/2 cup)
- 1 large bunch romaine lettuce or 1 (18-oz) package romaine hearts, coarsely chopped or torn and chilled

DIRECTIONS

FAST FIX

Prepare this entire recipe even if it's just for you! Store the dressing, chicken, and lettuce in separate containers in the refrigerator. Toss each serving together when you're ready to eat. The ingredients will keep in the refrigerator for 2 to 3 days.

1. Preheat the broiler. Pound the chicken with a kitchen mallet until it's about 1/2 inch thick. Rub the chicken with 1/2 tsp oil and sprinkle with 3/4 tsp pepper. Broil the chicken breasts on a baking pan for 8 minutes or until done, turning once. Let the cooked chicken rest for at least 5 minutes, then slice into thin (1/4-inch-wide) strips.

2. Add the jalapeño, garlic, cheese, mustard, Worcestershire sauce, tofu, and remaining black pepper to a blender and puree. Add the remaining oil and blend until smooth.

FRESH FACT

The spice is in the seeds and veins of the jalapeño, so remove them if you prefer mild dishes. For medium heat, simply use half a jalapeño—with seeds and veins. Just remember the heat from the jalapeño adds flavor, too, so go as spicy as you think you'll enjoy.

3. Before serving, toss dressing with the blackened chicken strips and lettuce. (If you toss while the chicken is hot, serve immediately so the lettuce doesn't wilt.) Alternatively, serve the dressing on the side so people can add their own. Serve with additional grated cheese, if desired.

Exchanges: 1 vegetable, 3 lean meat, 1/2 fat; 210 calories, 68 calories from fat, 8 g total fat, 2 g saturated fat, 70 mg cholesterol, 340 mg sodium, 7 g total carbohydrate, 3 g dietary fiber, 3 g sugars, 29 g protein.

FOOD FLAIR

There's no salt used in this salad. Think you need it? Don't automatically reach for the shaker. Instead, increase saltiness along with interesting flavor and extra nutrients by adding 4 anchovy filets to the blender when pureeing the dressing. Garnish with anchovy filets, too.

MORE THAN FOUR?

Toss the salad tableside (no more than 4 servings at a time) to impress your guests. For most vegetarians, simply toss in a separate bowl and serve their portion without chicken. (You'll need to use vegetarian Worcestershire sauce for the dressing, too.) For added taste excitement with or without chicken, toss every 4 servings with 1 cup large homemade-style croutons or 2 Tbsp roasted sunflower seeds.

MESCLUN SALAD WITH BOSC PEARS, PECANS, AND BLUE CHEESE

Serves 4/serving size: 2 1/2 cups

This perky salad is loaded with plenty of health-protective antioxidants from fresh fruit and nuts. Its pureed pear dressing is thick, tangy, and pink. No worries, guys will love it, too—pink dressing and all.

- 1/4 cup apple cider vinegar
- 1 1/2 Tbsp canola or flaxseed oil
- 2 medium Bosc pears, cored (divided use)
- 1/2 cup thinly sliced red onion (divided use)
- 1/2 tsp sea salt, or to taste
- 1/4 tsp ground cayenne red pepper
- 8 oz mesclun mix or mixed baby greens
- 1 cup seedless red grapes
- 2 Tbsp finely crumbled Artisanal blue or Maytag blue cheese
- 2 Tbsp chopped pecans or walnuts, pan-toasted

DIRECTIONS

1. Puree the vinegar, oil, half a pear (sliced), 1/4 cup onion, salt, and red pepper in a blender until smooth.

2. Just before serving, thinly slice the remaining pears. In a large bowl, toss the mesclun, grapes, pears, and remaining onion with the dressing. Arrange on salad plates. Sprinkle with cheese and pecans.

Exchanges: 1 1/2 fruit, 1 vegetable, 1 1/2 fat; 190 calories, 84 calories from fat, 9 g total fat, 1 g saturated fat, 5 mg cholesterol, 370 mg sodium, 27 g total carbohydrate, 6 g dietary fiber, 17 g sugars, 4 g protein.

FRESH FACT

When you use a sharp, full-flavored cheese, you don't need much. In this recipe, try Artisanal Great Hill Blue. It's piquant and pairs perfectly with pears and pecans. In fact, a little bit of high-flavored, full-fat cheese will be more satisfying than a lot of flavor-lacking, low-fat cheese. And when you just use a few crumbles of it, the recipe's total fat and saturated fat counts can still fit easily into nutritional guidelines for people with diabetes.

FOOD FLAIR

Go for extra nuttiness by using pecan oil in place of part or all of the canola or peanut oil. And whichever oil you choose to use in the recipe, consider serving the dressing on the side. That's so its lovely pink color is in the spotlight—and so everyone can add his or her desired amount. This salad is so tasty as it is, you might decide you want to enjoy it with less dressing, not more.

ROMAINE PEPPERCORN STEAK SALAD

Serves 4/serving size: 3 1/2 cups

This highly spiced entrée salad recipe was inspired by one I always enjoy when visiting Chicago's Gibsons Steakhouse. My cousin Monica and I often share their extra-large helping. Since I get a craving for it more often than I travel to the windy city, I made my own healthier version that's sized just right. Here it is.

- 1 large bunch romaine lettuce, coarsely chopped
- 1 (5-oz) package organic baby arugula or 1 bunch fresh arugula
- 1 1/2 cups thinly sliced red onion
- 2 Tbsp black peppercorns
- 2 (6-oz) lean beef tenderloin steaks (antibiotic free), about 1 1/4 inches thick
- 1/4 tsp sea salt, or to taste
- 1 pint grape tomatoes
- 1/3 cup natural low-fat or fat-free balsamic vinaigrette dressing
- 2 Tbsp finely crumbled feta cheese

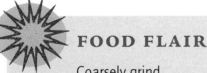

FOOD FLAIR

Coarsely grind different colors of peppercorns to rub or press on the steaks.

DIRECTIONS

1. In a large bowl, combine the lettuce, arugula, and onion. Keep chilled.

2. Coarsely grind the peppercorns in a spice or coffee grinder, peppermill, or food processor. Rub the peppercorns over both sides of steaks. Or pour the coarsely ground peppercorns onto a plate and firmly press both sides of each steak into them until coated. Lightly coat steaks with natural cooking spray.

FRESH FACT

Two terms that indicate leanness in beef are "loin" and "round." Lucky for lovers of tender, succulent beef, tenderloin is in that category. Besides being healthful, lean steak has a benefit in the skillet, too. Excess fat on steak can create significant smoke in your kitchen during medium-high- or high-temperature cooking. That's just one more reason to go lean.

3. Heat a large nonstick skillet over medium-high heat. Add the steaks and cook 4 minutes per side for medium rare. (Use your kitchen exhaust fan if steaks begin to smoke.) Sprinkle steaks with salt and let sit at least 5 minutes before slicing.

4. Meanwhile, toss the salad mixture with tomatoes and dressing. Arrange salad evenly on 4 plates. Slice each steak into 10 pieces. Serve steak on top of the salad and sprinkle with cheese.

Exchanges: 1/2 carbohydrate, 2 vegetable, 2 lean meat; 200 calories, 62 calories from fat, 7 g total fat, 2 g saturated fat, 45 mg cholesterol, 480 mg sodium, 19 g total carbohydrate, 6 g dietary fiber, 7 g sugars, 20 g protein.

MORE THAN FOUR?

Prep double or triple the amounts of all ingredients in advance. Coat the steaks with the peppercorn mixture up to 4 hours in advance. Cover and refrigerate. Up to 1 hour in advance of the meal, prepare the steaks until just barely medium rare. Then loosely cover with foil and place in a 200°F oven to continue cooking slightly more and keep warm until serving time. Toss the salad and slice the meat just before serving.

SPA CHEF SALAD WITH BALSAMIC TARRAGON DRESSING

Serves 4/serving size: 1/4 recipe

The magic to this entrée salad is the dressing. It's velvety from beans, zippy from vinegar and garlic, and extra fresh from tarragon. The creaminess from the beans will fool your taste buds into thinking this dressing is totally devilish, rather than wonderfully nutritious.

- 1 (15-oz) can organic no-salt-added white cannellini beans, drained (divided use)
- 1/4 cup aged balsamic vinegar
- 2 Tbsp extra virgin olive oil
- 2 large garlic cloves, peeled
- 1 Tbsp packed fresh tarragon leaves
- 1/4 tsp sea salt, or to taste
- 1 (5-oz) package mesclun salad blend
- 8 oz natural reduced-sodium smoked or oven-roasted turkey deli slices, cut into 1/3-inch strips
- 1 1/2 cups cherry tomatoes, halved
- 1 cup thinly sliced red onion

DIRECTIONS

1. Puree 1/2 cup beans, vinegar, oil, garlic, tarragon, and salt in a blender until smooth.

2. Arrange the mesclun on a large platter, then top with the turkey, tomatoes, onion, and remaining beans.

3. Garnish with additional fresh tarragon, if desired. Serve with dressing on the side (about 2 1/2 Tbsp per person).

Exchanges: 1 starch, 1 vegetable, 1 lean meat, 1 fat; 200 calories, 70 calories from fat, 8 g total fat, 1 g saturated fat, 25 mg cholesterol, 530 mg sodium, 17 g total carbohydrate, 4 g dietary fiber, 5 g sugars, 14 g protein.

FRESH FACT

Balsamic vinegar is usually made from white Trebbiano grape juice. It becomes darker and sharply sweeter as it's aged in wooden barrels. That enhances the umami (the "fifth taste") in the vinegar. And that means the older, the better. The splurge is well worth it! Look for balsamic vinegar aged 12 or more years . . . but vinegar that is aged 8 to 10 years is full of flavor, too.

ITALIAN CANNELLINI BEAN SALAD

Serves 4/serving size: scant 1 cup

Beans are packed with antioxidants. So while you're enjoying this fabulous salad full of freshness and texture, you're protecting your health, too. But it's the flavor that'll keep you coming back for more.

- 2 Tbsp aged red wine vinegar
- 1 Tbsp extra virgin olive oil
- 1 (15-oz) can organic no-salt-added white cannellini beans, drained
- 1/4 cup finely diced red onion
- 1 large vine-ripened tomato, seeded and diced (1 1/2 cups)
- 1/4 cup finely chopped fresh basil leaves, or mixture of basil and flat-leaf parsley
- 3 Tbsp finely diced celery
- 1/4 tsp sea salt, or to taste

DIRECTIONS

1. In a medium bowl, whisk the vinegar and oil.

2. Stir in the remaining ingredients and let the salad stand at least 20 minutes. Stir and serve at room temperature.

Exchanges: 1 starch, 1/2 fat; 100 calories, 37 calories from fat, 4 g total fat, 1 g saturated fat, 0 mg cholesterol, 170 mg sodium, 12 g total carbohydrate, 4 g dietary fiber, 3 g sugars, 4 g protein.

FRESH FACT

The best way to chop basil is to stack several leaves together, roll up tightly, and thinly slice crosswise. This is called "chiffonade." Make sure the basil leaves are dry when you slice them, as they can bruise when wet. Make sure you use a sharp knife, too.

FOOD FLAIR

If you want to take the time to soak and cook beans, try a variety of heirloom beans. Zolfini, Diavoli, and Pavoni are a few types to enjoy in this recipe.

MAYAN BEAN SALAD WITH FRESH CHILI–LIME VINAIGRETTE

Serves 4/serving size: 3/4 cup

Corn was a favorite food of the Mayan Indian. Eaten at every meal, it formed the backbone of Mayan cuisine. Another favorite was boiled black beans. Here they're beautifully married with fresh vinaigrette to create a salad that can double as a salsa. It's an appealing accompaniment to grilled chicken or fish, too.

- 1 serrano pepper or small jalapeño pepper, with seeds
- 1 large garlic clove
- 2 Tbsp lime juice
- 1 Tbsp extra virgin olive oil
- 1/4 tsp sea salt, or to taste
- 1 cup grape tomatoes, halved vertically
- 1 (15-oz) can organic black beans, well drained
- 2 (7-inch) ears yellow corn, grilled or pan-grilled, kernels cut off (see Fresh Fact)
- 1/4 cup finely diced red onion
- 2 Tbsp finely chopped fresh cilantro

DIRECTIONS

1. Puree the pepper, garlic, lime juice, oil, and salt in a blender. In a medium bowl, combine the tomatoes, beans, corn, onion, and cilantro. Drizzle with the vinaigrette and gently toss.

2. Let the salad stand at least 20 minutes to allow flavors to mingle. Stir and serve at room temperature. Garnish each serving with a fresh cilantro sprig, if desired.

Exchanges: 1 starch, 1 vegetable, 1/2 fat; 130 calories, 37 calories from fat, 4 g total fat, 1 g saturated fat, 0 mg cholesterol, 210 mg sodium, 20 g total carbohydrate, 4 g dietary fiber, 5 g sugars, 5 g protein.

FRESH FACT

To grill or pan-grill corn, lightly coat it with natural cooking spray or rub it very lightly with olive oil. Prepare a grill (use medium-high heat) and grill corn away from direct heat, rotating frequently, for 8 minutes, or until it's slightly blackened in spots. Or, place the corn in a nonstick pan over medium-high heat and cook for 8 minutes, rotating occasionally, until the corn is slightly blackened in spots and cooked through.

FAST FIX

When fresh corn is out of season or you simply want a quick fix, use 1 cup organic frozen or canned, drained corn—no grilling required.

MORE THAN FOUR?

This bean salad is good the next day—maybe better. That makes it a popular party food, since you don't need to worry about preparing it on party day. The recipe easily doubles, too.

FRESH FACT

When you hear that dry beans are good for your health, this includes canned beans, too. By choosing organic canned varieties, you'll be getting as close to nature as you can without soaking the dry beans yourself. Plus, using canned beans saves a lot of time. If sodium is a concern for you, buy canned beans with no added salt, or rinse them to reduce up to 50% of the sodium.

VALENCIA ORANGE BULGUR SALAD WITH ALMONDS AND FRESH MINT

Serves 6/serving size: rounded 1 cup

Mediterranean fare is traditionally diabetes-friendly. It's filled with farm-fresh produce, nuts, and olive oil—all of which are part of this salad. But since most of us can't just jump up and go to Greece, Italy, or Spain, preparing this Mediterranean-inspired salad can bring some of the healthful pleasures of their cuisine to our tables.

- 1 1/4 cups freshly squeezed Valencia or other orange juice
- 1 cup bulgur wheat
- 1 1/2 Tbsp extra virgin olive oil
- 2 1/2 cups diced yellow or white onion
- 2 large garlic cloves, minced
- 2 large vine-ripened tomatoes, seeded and diced (2 1/2 cups)
- 2/3 cup chopped, fresh flat-leaf parsley
- 1/3 cup chopped fresh mint
- 1 tsp sea salt, or to taste
- 3 Tbsp slivered almonds, pan-toasted

DIRECTIONS

1. Bring the orange juice to a simmer in a small saucepan over medium heat. Place the bulgur in a medium bowl and pour the simmering juice over bulgur.

2. Heat the oil in a large nonstick skillet over medium heat. Add the onion and cook, stirring, for 5 minutes or until the onion is softened. Add the garlic and cook, stirring, for 2 minutes (but don't let the garlic brown). Stir the mixture into the bulgur, cover, and refrigerate at least 45 minutes.

3. Just before serving, gently stir the tomatoes, parsley, mint, and salt into the bulgur. Sprinkle with almonds and serve at room temperature.

Exchanges: 1 1/2 starch, 1 vegetable, 1 fat; 190 calories, 53 calories from fat, 6 g total fat, 1 g saturated fat, 0 mg cholesterol, 400 mg sodium, 32 g total carbohydrate, 7 g dietary fiber, 8 g sugars, 5 g protein.

FRESH FACT

Bulgur, a whole grain, is made by parboiling, drying, and cracking whole grain wheat. And because that's already done for us when we buy it, you don't have to cook it at all—just soak it! Using water as the soaking liquid is fine . . . but stock or juice can provide extra flavor and health-protective nutrition.

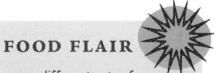

FOOD FLAIR

Did you know there are different cuts of bulgur? Visit a Mediterranean, Middle Eastern, or other international market whenever you get a chance to try all varieties. A popular choice, #2 bulgur, works best in this salad. It's a medium texture—not too fine and not too coarse.

CALIFORNIA AVOCADO–BEAN SALAD WITH SALSA VERDE

Serves 6/serving size: 1 cup

People with diabetes are sometimes reluctant to eat avocados. No worries, though: avocados may seem rich and buttery, but they're full of "good" fats and other health-protective ingredients, like folate and potassium. That makes the avocado a winner for people with diabetes—and for everyone. You'll see how delicious they can be in this zesty salad.

- 1 (15-oz) can organic black beans, well drained
- 1 (15-oz) can organic cannellini or other white beans, well drained
- 1 cup diced red onion
- 1 1/3 cups diced red or yellow bell pepper
- 1 large jalapeño pepper with or without seeds, minced (optional)
- 1/4 cup chopped fresh cilantro
- 2/3 cup commercially made tomatillo sauce (salsa verde), or see recipe, page 72
- 1 Hass avocado, peeled and diced
- 1/4 tsp sea salt, or to taste

DIRECTIONS

1. In a large bowl, combine the beans, onion, bell pepper, jalapeño (if using), and cilantro.

2. Stir in the tomatillo sauce. Then add the avocado and salt and stir gently. Serve as a salad.

Exchanges: 1 starch, 1 vegetable, 1 fat; 150 calories, 43 calories from fat, 5 g total fat, 1 g saturated fat, 0 mg cholesterol, 150 mg sodium, 22 g total carbohydrate, 6 g dietary fiber, 4 g sugars, 6 g protein.

FOOD FLAIR

You can also serve this in a bowl like salsa, with baked blue corn tortilla chips on the side. Or serve as an appetizer by placing a scoop of bean salad on top of a thick tomato slice. Also, consider using white corn or hominy in place of the white beans for a change of texture and taste. Or use a 2 1/2-cup three-bean mixture, such as black, cannellini, and red kidney beans, instead of just the two types.

FAST FIX

Skip the jalapeño if you're using spicy tomatillo sauce. And when you use spicy sauce, start with 1/3 cup—then add more if you like more heat.

MORE THAN FOUR?

Go ahead and double this recipe. Wait until just before serving to dice and gently stir in the avocado. But if you can't wait, toss the diced avocado with lime juice or a mixture of lime and lemon juice. That way, it'll be less likely to turn brown.

NEW-AGE NIÇOISE SALAD WITH GRAPE TOMATOES AND LEMON–BASIL VINAIGRETTE

Serves 4/serving size: 1/4 recipe

This French-inspired entrée salad is gorgeous. Best of all, it's so satisfying that you'll find it hard to believe a serving has less than 200 calories.

- 1/4 cup lemon juice
- 2 Tbsp extra virgin olive oil or garlic-flavored olive oil
- 1/4 tsp garlic salt, or to taste
- 1/4 cup finely chopped fresh basil leaves

- 3 cups organic baby arugula or baby spinach
- 1 pint grape tomatoes
- 1 1/2 cups sliced English (hothouse) cucumber with skin

- 2 large hard-boiled eggs, quartered
- 1 (7-oz) can water-packed solid tuna, drained and separated into chunks
- 12 kalamata or other olives

DIRECTIONS

1. In a small bowl, whisk the lemon juice, oil, and garlic salt. Stir in the basil.

2. Arrange a bed of arugula or spinach on a large platter. Arrange the tomatoes, cucumbers, eggs, tuna, and olives on top of the greens. Drizzle with vinaigrette. Sprinkle salad with additional garlic salt (optional).

Exchanges: 1 vegetable, 2 lean meat, 1 fat; 190 calories, 103 calories from fat, 11 g total fat, 2 g saturated fat, 120 mg cholesterol, 370 mg sodium, 7 g total carbohydrate, 2 g dietary fiber, 3 g sugars, 15 g protein.

FRESH FACT

If you prefer one of the tuna brands that come in 6-oz cans instead of 7, go ahead and use it—and toss on a few extra olives. But before you use the tuna, read the ingredient label. Some commercial brands contain broth and an additive, pyrophosphate. Your best tuna bet is usually to choose a less commercial brand that has the truest fish flavors, natural juices, and healthful oils. Look for a brand that has just tuna (usually yellowfin tuna), water, and salt.

FOOD FLAIR

Sprinkle fresh tarragon or thinly sliced green onion on the salad. For a salty kick, top it with anchovies. And for garlic lovers, stir a large minced garlic clove into the vinaigrette.

LEMONY MEDITERRANEAN EGGPLANT SALAD WITH BASIL AND PINE NUTS

Serves 4/serving size: 3/4 cup

The glossy, dark purple-skinned eggplant is freshest in August and September, when it's in season. So make this salad a staple at your Labor Day festivities. Use this recipe to experiment with various types of eggplant, including Japanese, Chinese, Italian, baby, or white.

- 1 medium eggplant with skin, stem removed and sliced lengthwise into 4 strips
- 2 Tbsp lemon juice
- 2 large shallots, thinly sliced
- 1 Tbsp extra virgin olive oil
- 1/2 tsp sea salt, or to taste
- 1/3 cup thinly sliced fresh basil leaves
- 2 Tbsp pan-toasted pine nuts

DIRECTIONS

1. Heat the grill over medium-high heat. Grill the eggplant 4 to 5 minutes per side or until lightly charred and cooked through. Meanwhile, combine the lemon juice, shallots, oil, and salt in a medium bowl.

2. Cut each grilled eggplant slice into large bite-size pieces. Toss the eggplant with the dressing until just coated. Just before serving, stir in basil and top with pine nuts. Serve cool or at room temperature.

Exchanges: 2 vegetable, 1 fat; 90 calories, 59 calories from fat, 7 g total fat, 1 g saturated fat, 0 mg cholesterol, 290 mg sodium, 8 g total carbohydrate, 3 g dietary fiber, 4 g sugars, 2 g protein.

FOOD FLAIR

Roasted eggplant has a different flavor than grilled, but cooked in either style, eggplant is memorable. To roast, wrap the whole eggplant in foil. Place on a rack in a 400°F oven for 35 to 40 minutes or until thoroughly cooked. Chill. Cut off the stem of cool eggplant, then cut into large bite-size pieces.

FAST FIX

Too cold to cook outdoors? Place a grill pan over medium-high heat. Once hot, add eggplant in batches. Cook 4 minutes per side or until done. Or in a panini-style indoor grill on medium-high heat, grill eggplant in batches, 5 to 6 minutes total, or until done.

FRESH HERB QUINOA TABBOULEH

Serves 4/serving size: 1 cup

Tabbouleh is a Middle Eastern grain salad that's traditionally made with bulgur wheat. Here, it's updated using the highly nutritious, naturally quick-cooking whole grain, quinoa.

- 1 1/2 cups spring water
- 3/4 cup quinoa
- 2 Tbsp lemon juice
- 1 Tbsp extra virgin olive oil
- 1 large vine-ripened tomato, seeded and diced (1 1/2 cups)
- 1/3 cup thinly sliced green onion
- 1/3 cup chopped fresh flat-leaf parsley
- 1/4 cup finely diced English (hothouse) cucumber with skin
- 1/4 cup chopped fresh mint
- 3/4 tsp garlic salt
- 1/4 tsp freshly ground black pepper, or to taste

DIRECTIONS

1. Bring the water and quinoa to a boil in a medium saucepan over high heat. Reduce the heat to medium, cover, and simmer for 10 minutes. Remove from heat and let sit for 5 minutes, covered. Transfer to a medium bowl and chill.

2. Meanwhile, in a small bowl, whisk the lemon juice and oil in a medium bowl. Stir in the tomato, green onion, parsley, cucumber, and mint. Stir this mixture into the chilled quinoa, then add the garlic salt and pepper.

3. Use a slotted spoon for serving to drain off any excess liquid. Serve at room temperature.

Exchanges: 1 1/2 starch, 1 vegetable, 1 fat; 170 calories, 50 calories from fat, 6 g total fat, 1 g saturated fat, 0 mg cholesterol, 200 mg sodium, 27 g total carbohydrate, 3 g dietary fiber, 2 g sugars, 5 g protein.

FRESH FACT

If you prefer the taste of fresh garlic, use 1 large minced garlic clove and 1/4 tsp sea salt in place of 3/4 tsp garlic salt. I personally prefer using this fresh garlic and sea salt option. However, in this and a few other recipes in this cookbook, I suggest using garlic salt as a timesaver—and when overall flavors are not negatively affected.

FAST FIX

Step 1 can be done up to 2 days in advance. Keep covered and refrigerated until ready to use.

FOOD FLAIR

Think of tabbouleh as more than just salad. Stuff it into whole grain pita halves and enjoy as a sandwich. Mound it into hollowed-out tomato halves, and serve as an appetizer. Be creative.

BOW TIE MACARONI SALAD

Serves 6/serving size: 1 cup

Looking for a perky picnic or cool cookout salad or side that's healthful, too? Look no further. By adding lean ham, this modern macaroni salad will provide protein to help balance its carbs. Enjoy it with lean grilled steak, pork, or chicken to help keep the total carbohydrates in your outdoor meal deliciously in check.

- 8 oz dry farfalle (bow tie) or fusilli pasta, regular or whole wheat (3 1/2 cups dry)
- 3 Tbsp mayonnaise
- 2 Tbsp apple cider vinegar
- 1/4 tsp paprika
- 1/4 tsp hot pepper sauce
- 5 oz natural lean baked or smoked ham, diced
- 4 oz jarred, drained, roasted red bell pepper, chopped (2/3 cup)
- 1/3 cup thinly sliced green onion
- 8 cornichons (midget gherkins), very thinly sliced horizontally

DIRECTIONS

1. Cook the pasta according to package directions, omitting added oil and salt. Drain and gently rinse with cold water to cool quickly. Drain well.

2. Meanwhile, in a small bowl, whisk the mayonnaise, vinegar, paprika, and pepper sauce. Chill.

3. In a large bowl, combine the ham, bell pepper, green onion, and cornichons with the pasta. Just before serving, add the dressing and toss.

Exchanges: 2 1/2 starch, 1 lean meat, 1/2 fat; 260 calories, 67 calories from fat, 7 g total fat, 1 g saturated fat, 15 mg cholesterol, 550 mg sodium, 34 g total carbohydrate, 1 g dietary fiber, 3 g sugars, 11 g protein.

FRESH FACTS

Cornichon is the French word for "gherkin." Cornichons are crisp, tart pickles made from tiny gherkin cucumbers. They're a traditional accompaniment to pâtés, as well as smoked fish and meats.

There's no need for low-fat or fat-free mayo. Use real mayo for full flavor, but use less of it. Then stretch it by thinning with vinegar to make a mayo-based sauce. That way it'll dress every piece of pasta—or anything else you want to toss with the sauce. But if you want a thicker mayo-based dressing, like for chicken, tuna, or potato salad, mix the mayo with fat-free plain yogurt or organic low-fat sour cream and a touch of Dijon mustard or hot pepper sauce to punch up the flavor. Have fun and experiment!

FOOD FLAIR

Use a freshly roasted or grilled red bell pepper instead of the jarred variety, for a fresh-roasted or outdoor-grilled flair. It'll reduce the sodium in this recipe, too—to 400 mg per serving.

FAST FIX

Cook pasta a day in advance—but don't rinse with water. Instead, toss with 2 tsp canola oil so the pasta doesn't stick together. Cover and chill. Make the mayonnaise sauce mixture in advance, too. Cover and chill. Start with Step 3 the next day, right before you're ready to serve.

SOUTHERN BLACK-EYED PEA SALAD

Serves 4/serving size: 3/4 cup

Get a taste of the South … with a good kick! You'll love the textures, colors and, of course, all the great flavors. To top that off, this sensational legume salad is rich in vitamin C and fiber.

- 1 (15.5-oz) can organic black-eyed peas, drained, or 1 1/2 cups cooked, chilled black-eyed peas
- 1/2 cup diced celery
- 1/2 cup diced red bell pepper
- 1/2 cup diced white or red onion
- 2 Tbsp apple cider vinegar
- 1 1/2 Tbsp extra virgin olive or canola oil
- 1 Tbsp wildflower or clover honey
- 1 large garlic clove, minced
- 1 small jalapeño pepper with some seeds, minced
- 1/2 tsp sea salt, or to taste

DIRECTIONS

1. In a large bowl, combine the black-eyed peas, celery, bell pepper, and onion. In a small bowl, whisk the vinegar, oil, honey, garlic, jalapeño, and salt.

2. Pour the dressing over the black-eyed peas and stir. If possible, refrigerate overnight to let the flavors marry. Stir before serving.

FOOD FLAIR

Stir in diced low-sodium ham before serving to create a more savory side—or a delicious entrée, too.

Exchanges: 1 1/2 carbohydrate, 1 fat; 150 calories, 55 calories from fat, 6 g total fat, 1 g saturated fat, 0 mg cholesterol, 320 mg sodium, 20 g total carbohydrate, 4 g dietary fiber, 7 g sugars, 5 g protein.

BOWLFUL

AMERICAN–FRENCH CARAMELIZED ONION SOUP

Serves 4/serving size: 1 2/3 cups

Browning onions makes them sweeter—and it makes sweet onions sweeter yet. The result: a soup loaded with onions in a beautiful balance of savory and sweet.

- 1 Tbsp extra virgin olive oil
- 3 large Vidalia, Maui, or other sweet onions, very thinly sliced (8 cups)
- 2 large garlic cloves, minced
- 2 tsp minced fresh thyme leaves
- 4 cups natural fat-free chicken broth
- 1 tsp unsalted butter
- 1/2 tsp freshly ground pepper, or to taste
- 1/4 tsp hot pepper sauce, or to taste
- 1/8 tsp sea salt, or to taste

DIRECTIONS

1. Heat the oil in a stockpot or extra-large saucepan over medium heat. Add onions and cook, stirring occasionally, for 10 minutes. Increase the heat to medium high. Cook, stirring occasionally, for 10 minutes more, or until all the onions turn a caramel color.

2. Add the garlic and thyme and cook another 2 minutes. Add the chicken broth and increase the heat to high. Bring just to a boil while scraping up and stirring into the broth any browned bits from the pot. Stir in the butter and remove from the heat. Add pepper, pepper sauce, and salt.

Exchanges: 2 carbohydrate, 1 fat; 190 calories, 43 calories from fat, 5 g total fat, 1 g saturated fat, 5 mg cholesterol, 470 mg sodium, 29 g total carbohydrate, 5 g dietary fiber, 13 g sugars, 8 g protein.

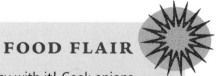

FOOD FLAIR

Use this recipe as a starting point. Then play with it! Cook onions until they're a dark caramel color rather than light—the soup will be richer and sweeter. Try beef-flavored broth instead of chicken. Use a variety of onions, like red, yellow, and sweet, so the soup is more savory. Add more broth so it can easily serve 6 or 8 rather than 4. Serve each bowl topped with a small piece of toasted whole grain bread covered with melted Gruyère or another Swiss cheese.

CARROT–GINGER POTAGE

Serves 4/serving size: 1 2/3 cups

Potage is a French term for a thick soup. This vivid pureed potage is thick from healthful vegetables, not added cream.

- 2 tsp unsalted butter
- 1 lb baby carrots
- 1/2 cup sliced celery
- 1 1/2 cups sliced yellow onion
- 1 Tbsp grated fresh ginger
- 2 medium Yukon gold potatoes, peeled and sliced
- 5 cups spring water
- 1/2 tsp sea salt, or to taste
- 1/4 tsp hot pepper sauce, or to taste

DIRECTIONS

1. Melt the butter in a stockpot or extra-large saucepan over medium heat. Sauté the carrots, celery, onion, and ginger for 5 minutes.

2. Increase the heat to high and add the potatoes, water, and salt. Bring to a boil. Reduce the heat to medium and simmer, uncovered, for 25 minutes, or until the potatoes and carrots are very tender.

3. Use a hand blender to puree the soup in the pot. Or puree the soup in batches in a blender, reheating in a clean pot over medium heat. (See the "hot fill" line on your blender container for guidance, if available.) Add hot pepper sauce to taste and serve hot.

FOOD FLAIR

Potatoes, not cream, add the thick richness to this soup. You could also stir in evaporated fat-free milk after pureeing to create a thinner, yet creamier soup. For an eye-appealing finale, serve topped with minced green onions or chives.

Exchanges: 1 starch, 2 vegetable, 1/2 fat; 150 calories, 19 calories from fat, 2 g total fat, 1 g saturated fat, 5 mg cholesterol, 390 mg sodium, 30 g total carbohydrate, 6 g dietary fiber, 8 g sugars, 3 g protein.

LEMON-ZESTED WHITE BEAN AND ESCAROLE SOUP

Serves 4/serving size: 1 1/2 cups

Wow, a hot soup that's actually refreshing! It'll provide you with a clever way to sneak some beans into your meals, too. And that's always a good thing since the soluble fiber in beans helps with blood glucose and blood cholesterol management.

- 1 Tbsp extra virgin olive oil
- 3/4 cup thinly sliced white onion
- 2 cups firmly packed shredded escarole
- 1 large garlic clove, minced
- 4 cups natural fat-free chicken broth
- 1 (15.5-oz) can organic cannellini or other white beans, drained
- 2 tsp lemon zest (grated peel), or to taste
- 1/8 tsp hot pepper sauce, or to taste

DIRECTIONS

1. Heat the oil in a large saucepan over medium heat. Sauté the onion for 3 minutes. Add the escarole and garlic and sauté 2 minutes.

2. Add the broth and beans. Increase the heat to high and bring just to a boil. Remove from the heat and add lemon zest and hot pepper sauce to taste. Garnish with additional lemon zest, if desired.

Exchanges: 1 carbohydrate, 1 lean meat; 130 calories, 37 calories from fat, 4 g total fat, 1 g saturated fat, 0 mg cholesterol, 410 mg sodium, 14 g total carbohydrate, 4 g dietary fiber, 2 g sugars, 9 g protein.

FRESH FACT

It's the aromatic oils from the lemon zest that add much flavor. By using zest, you can use less of the rest. That means added salt isn't necessary in this lovely soup.

LEEK AND POTATO CHOWDER

Serves 4/serving size: 1 1/4 cups

This might be the first chowder you can feel good about chowing down. It tastes devilishly rich. And in fact, it is devilishly rich—in nutrition.

- 1 Tbsp extra virgin olive oil
- 4 medium leeks, white and light green parts only, thinly sliced
- 2 medium Yukon gold potatoes, peeled and diced (2 cups)
- 2 cups natural fat-free chicken or vegetable broth
- 1/2 tsp ground sage
- 3 Tbsp unbleached all-purpose flour
- 2 cups fat-free milk (divided use)
- 1/4 cup chopped fresh flat-leaf parsley
- 1/4 tsp sea salt, or to taste
- 2 Tbsp minced fresh chives

DIRECTIONS

1. Heat the oil in a large saucepan over medium heat. Sauté the leeks for 5 minutes or until softened.

2. Increase the heat to medium high. Add the potatoes, broth, and sage. Cover and cook 8 minutes or until the potatoes are nearly tender.

3. Whisk the flour with 1/4 cup milk until smooth. Stir it, along with the remaining milk, into the potato–leek mixture. Heat, uncovered, for 5 minutes or until slightly thickened and potatoes are tender, stirring occasionally.

4. Remove from the heat and stir in the parsley and salt. Sprinkle with chives to serve.

Exchanges: 1 1/2 starch, 1/2 fat-free milk, 1 vegetable, 1/2 fat; 210 calories, 34 calories from fat, 4 g total fat, 1 g saturated fat, 0 mg cholesterol, 420 mg sodium, 35 g total carbohydrate, 3 g dietary fiber, 10 g sugars, 10 g protein.

FRESH FACT

Leeks are most lovable from October through May. But whenever you buy them, they're only lovable if you get out the grit. For this chowder, clean the leeks by slicing vertically once, then thinly slicing horizontally. Add them to a bowl of water, swish around, rinse, and drain well before using.

FOOD FLAIR

You can forgo the flour if you like. If you do, increase the cooking time in Step 3 another 5 or more minutes. Instead of flour acting as a thickener, the natural starch from the potatoes will do the job—plus the extra cooking time will reduce the liquid a bit. If you like, mash the mixture to create an even thicker soup. And for added texture and taste, sprinkle each serving with natural bacon bits along with the chives.

FAST FIX

Make good use of your time when preparing this chowder. While the potatoes are cooking in the broth, gather, measure, and prep the remaining ingredients, beginning with the flour.

JALAPEÑO CORN CHOWDER

Serves 4/serving size: 1 1/4 cups

Though there's no cream in this good-for-you chowder, it's surprisingly decadent—and creamy. And though savory, it has a wonderful natural sweetness from the bell pepper, corn, and evaporated milk. Just be sure to pair this carb-rich soup with a protein-packed entrée—try roasted chicken breast or grilled lean flank steak seasoned with cumin and cilantro—to create a balanced, diabetes-friendly meal.

- 2 tsp unsalted butter
- 1 cup diced white onion
- 1 cup diced red bell pepper
- 1 jalapeño pepper with some seeds, halved vertically and thinly sliced crosswise
- 1/2 tsp ground cumin
- 3 Tbsp unbleached all-purpose flour
- 1 1/2 cups natural fat-free chicken broth
- 1 cup evaporated fat-free milk
- 1 lb frozen whole yellow corn, thawed
- 2 Tbsp finely chopped fresh cilantro

DIRECTIONS

1. Melt the butter in a large saucepan over medium heat. Add the onion, bell pepper, jalapeño, and cumin. Cook, stirring, for 10 minutes or until the onion and peppers are tender.

2. Add the flour and stir 1 minute. Vigorously stir in the broth and evaporated milk. Increase the heat to high and bring to a boil while stirring. Add the corn and cook for 2 minutes. Top with cilantro to serve.

Exchanges: 3 carbohydrate; 220 calories, 25 calories from fat, 3 g total fat, 1 g saturated fat, 5 mg cholesterol, 230 mg sodium, 41 g total carbohydrate, 4 g dietary fiber, 15 g sugars, 10 g protein.

FRESH FACT

Evaporated milk is regular milk with 60% of the water removed. Since it has less water, it provides a wonderful, creamy texture. It's a bit sweeter than regular milk, but has no added sugar. The slight sweetness comes from the natural sugar in milk—lactose.

FAST FIX

Place the frozen corn in a bowl in the refrigerator in the morning—it'll thaw by dinnertime.

PUREE OF BROCCOLI SOUP WITH FRESHLY GRATED NUTMEG

Serves 4/serving size: scant 1 cup

Nutmeg is considered a sweet spice that's lovely in this broccoli soup. And when you add freshly grated nutmeg from the whole spice just before serving—rather than ground nutmeg from a year-old spice bottle—you won't believe how its aromatic, warm, sweet, and spicy essence takes this soup from ordinary to extraordinary.

- 2 tsp unsalted butter
- 3/4 cup chopped white onion
- 1/4 tsp white pepper
- 4 cups bite-size broccoli florets and tender stems
- 3 cups natural fat-free chicken broth
- 2 tsp fresh lemon juice
- 1/2 cup fat-free evaporated milk
- 1/8 tsp freshly grated or ground nutmeg
- 1/8 tsp sea salt, or to taste

DIRECTIONS

1. Melt the butter in a large saucepan over medium heat. Sauté the onion and white pepper for 3 minutes or until the onion is softened.

2. Add the broccoli, broth, and lemon juice. Simmer, covered, for 20 minutes or until the broccoli is very tender.

3. Use a hand blender to puree the soup in the pot. Or puree the soup in batches in a blender, reheating in a clean pot over medium heat. (See the "hot fill" line on your blender container for guidance, if available.)

4. Stir in the evaporated milk, nutmeg, and salt. Heat the soup for 3 minutes or until hot.

Exchanges: 1 carbohydrate, 1/2 fat; 100 calories, 20 calories from fat, 2 g total fat, 1 g saturated fat, 5 mg cholesterol, 430 mg sodium, 14 g total carbohydrate, 3 g dietary fiber, 7 g sugars, 8 g protein.

FRESH FACT

To freshly grate nutmeg from the whole spice, first buy the jar of whole spice next to the ground nutmeg jar in the spice aisle, then grate! It couldn't be easier to add extra flavor to all your recipes calling for nutmeg.

FOOD FLAIR

Serve this soup as a sauce over plain ol' chicken 'n' rice. Wow, that's nice.

CREAMY CHESTNUT SOUP

Serves 4/serving size: 1 cup

It's rare to find a soup that's so thick, creamy, and intriguing. Serve it at Thanksgiving to add a gourmet touch to your tradition. Or serve it with any routine meal to make it brilliant.

- 2 (7.4-oz) jars vacuum-packed chestnuts
- 3 1/2 cups natural fat-free chicken or vegetable broth
- 1 rounded cup chopped Vidalia, Maui, or other sweet onion
- Pinch allspice
- 2 bay leaves
- 1/2 cup plain soy milk
- 1 tsp turbinado sugar
- 1/8 tsp sea salt, or to taste
- 1/4 tsp freshly ground white pepper, or to taste
- 2 Tbsp finely chopped fresh flat-leaf parsley (optional)

DIRECTIONS

1. Bring the chestnuts, broth, onion, allspice, and bay leaves to a boil in a large saucepan over high heat. Reduce the heat to medium and simmer, uncovered, for 15 minutes. Remove the bay leaves.

2. Use a hand blender to puree the soup in the pot. Or puree the soup in batches in a blender, reheating in a clean pot over medium heat. (See the "hot fill" line on your blender container for guidance, if available.)

3. Stir in the soy milk, sugar, salt, and pepper and gently heat through. Top with parsley to serve (if using).

Exchanges: 2 1/2 carbohydrate, 1/2 fat; 210 calories, 19 calories from fat, 2 g total fat, 0 g saturated fat, 0 mg cholesterol, 450 mg sodium, 39 g total carbohydrate, 2 g dietary fiber, 5 g sugars, 8 g protein.

FAST FIX

Instead of making a soup and gravy, just make this recipe. It doubles as gravy for turkey or mashed potatoes. It's a delightfully surprising addition to a holiday meal—or an anyday meal.

MORE THAN FOUR?

Preparing this soup for a big family gathering or a party? Instead of passing the salt and pepper, pass around a small bowl of turbinado sugar! Your guests can sweeten their servings to create their own perfect sweet-savory balance.

SECRET INGREDIENT SERRANO CHILI CON CARNE

Serves 4/serving size: 1 1/4 cups

Finally, a chili that's as pleasing for football-watching males as it is for figure-watching females—and vice versa. It tastes like it's been slow-simmered for hours. Fix it for fun family dinners or friendly gatherings. Or just make it for yourself—for your next four meals. It's that good—and that good for you.

- 1 lb lean ground beef sirloin (antibiotic free)
- 2 cups chopped red onion
- 2 large garlic cloves, minced
- 1 serrano pepper with seeds, minced
- 3 Tbsp chili powder
- 1 tsp ground cinnamon
- 1 (14.25-oz) can natural fat-free beef-flavored broth
- 3/4 cup canned organic crushed tomatoes
- 1 (15.5-oz) can organic black beans, drained
- 1/4 tsp sea salt, or to taste
- 1/4 cup chopped fresh cilantro (divided use; optional)

DIRECTIONS

1. Heat a stockpot or large saucepan over medium-high heat. Add the beef, onion, garlic, and serrano pepper. Sauté 5 minutes or until the meat is cooked through and the onions are softened. Add the chili powder and cinnamon and sauté 1 minute.

2. Add the broth and tomatoes and reduce the heat to medium. Partially cover and simmer 20 minutes or until the chili is thick, stirring occasionally. Stir in the beans, salt, and 2 Tbsp cilantro (if using). Top with remaining cilantro to serve.

Exchanges: 1 1/2 carbohydrate, 3 lean meat; 260 calories, 51 calories from fat, 6 g total fat, 2 g saturated fat, 40 mg cholesterol, 560 mg sodium, 24 g total carbohydrate, 7 g dietary fiber, 5 g sugars, 29 g protein.

FOOD FLAIR

Go for two secret ingredients! The cinnamon was the first. Now add 1 tsp natural unsweetened cocoa powder. This is the secret (or not-so-secret) combination of flavors in Cincinnati chili. You can adjust the amounts of cinnamon and cocoa to your taste each time you make this recipe. Or, if you don't mind giving away one secret, serve each cup with a cinnamon stick.

FAST FIX

Make this a day ahead, cover, and refrigerate. Then reheat over medium heat the next day while you're watching the game.

MORE THAN FOUR?

As a salute to San Francisco, serve this chili in hollowed-out sourdough bread rounds. These edible bowls will help make this chili hip, not just hot.

SPLIT PEA SOUP WITH NATURAL HAM

Serves 4/serving size: 3/4 cup

The most noted culinary role of split peas is in homey split pea soup. This version is a luscious, feel-good way to enjoy these legumes.

- 2 tsp extra virgin olive oil
- 1 cup diced white onion
- 12 baby carrots, cut horizontally into 1/4-inch coins
- 2 cups natural fat-free chicken broth
- 3 oz thick-cut natural lean baked or smoked ham, cut into 1/2-inch cubes
- 2 cups spring water
- 1/2 cup dry green split peas, rinsed
- 2 bay leaves
- 1/4 tsp freshly ground black pepper, or to taste
- 1/2 tsp chopped fresh thyme leaves

DIRECTIONS

1. Heat the oil in a stockpot or large saucepan over medium-high heat. Sauté the onion and carrots for 5 minutes or until the onions just begin to brown.

2. Add the broth, ham, water, split peas, bay leaves, and pepper. Increase the heat to high and bring to a boil. Reduce the heat to medium low and simmer, uncovered, stirring occasionally, for 1 hour and 10 minutes or until desired consistency.

3. Remove the bay leaves and stir in the thyme. Serve in mugs or small soup bowls.

FRESH FACT

Split peas are just field peas that are split and dried. They don't need soaking—just time to simmer.

Exchanges: 1 1/2 carbohydrate, 1 lean meat; 180 calories, 32 calories from fat, 4 g total fat, 1 g saturated fat, 10 mg cholesterol, 420 mg sodium, 23 g total carbohydrate, 2 g dietary fiber, 4 g sugars, 14 g protein.

CHILLY ORGANIC CUCUMBER SOUP WITH FRESH MINT

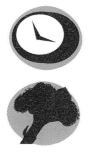

Serves 4/serving size: 3/4 cup

This soup is served chilled, making it an exceptionally refreshing palate-pleaser for spring or summertime. And it's a cool way to eat your veggies.

- 1 (12-inch) organic English (hothouse) cucumber with skin, sliced
- 1 cup natural vegetable broth
- 1/2 cup cultured reduced-fat buttermilk
- 1/4 tsp sea salt, or to taste
- 1/4 cup fresh mint leaves

DIRECTIONS

Puree the cucumber, broth, buttermilk, salt, and mint (reserving 4 leaves for garnish) in a blender until smooth. Garnish with mint leaves to serve.

Exchanges: 1 vegetable; 35 calories, 7 calories from fat, 1 g total fat, 0 g saturated fat, 0 mg cholesterol, 290 mg sodium, 5 g total carbohydrate, 1 g dietary fiber, 3 g sugars, 3 g protein.

FRESH FACT

Since the English cucumber, also known as a hothouse cucumber, is relatively seedless and thin-skinned, there's no need to peel it or remove its seeds. That makes it easier to use than a common American cucumber—and worth the extra expense. You'll probably find it tastes better, too.

VIETNAMESE-STYLE BEEF AND SOBA NOODLE SOUP

Serves 4/serving size: 1 cup

Serve this soup as an entrée along with chopsticks. Then slurp up the remaining broth. It's fun to eat—unless you're serving it on a first date or to a group of overly well-mannered people.

- 1/4 cup rice vinegar
- 2 Tbsp naturally brewed reduced-sodium soy sauce
- 2 large garlic cloves, minced
- 2 tsp toasted sesame oil
- 2 tsp acacia or other mild honey
- 2 tsp grated fresh ginger root
- 10 oz lean beef tenderloin (antibiotic free), cut into 1/4-inch strips
- 3 oz dry soba noodles
- 1 (14.25-oz) can natural fat-free beef-flavored broth
- 1/4 cup thinly sliced green onion
- 1/4 cup chopped fresh mint (optional)

DIRECTIONS

1. In a medium bowl, combine the vinegar, soy sauce, garlic, oil, honey, and ginger. Add the beef and toss to coat. Set aside to marinate up to 20 minutes.

2. Meanwhile, in a large saucepan, boil the soba noodles until tender, but still firm, about 4 minutes (or 1 minute less than package instructions). Drain.

3. In a large saucepan over high heat, bring the broth to a boil. Add the noodles and beef with marinade. Cook 2 minutes, or until a full boil is reached and the beef is cooked through. Top with green onion and mint (if using) to serve.

Exchanges: 1 1/2 carbohydrate, 2 lean meat; 220 calories, 58 calories from fat, 7 g total fat, 2 g saturated fat, 40 mg cholesterol, 560 mg sodium, 21 g total carbohydrate, 1 g dietary fiber, 3 g sugars, 21 g protein.

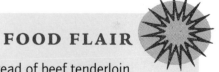

FOOD FLAIR

For a heartier soup, use flank steak instead of beef tenderloin. It's less pricy, but also less tender. Simply marinate the meat, covered, in the refrigerator for 2 hours to help tenderize it. Then move on to Step 2.

SIMMERED LAMB AND VEGETABLE STEW

Serves 4/serving size: scant 1 1/2 cups

Comfort food is oh-so-flavorful, yet often oh-so-fattening. But now you can have comfort food without the guilt. This rich stew is a satisfying entrée full of flavor. It's an enjoyable way to get extra veggies, too.

- 10 oz lean lamb shoulder without bone, cut into 1-inch cubes (antibiotic free)
- 1/4 cup unbleached, all-purpose flour
- 2 tsp extra virgin olive oil
- 1 3/4 cups sliced white onion
- 2 cups spring water
- 1 1/4 cups canned organic crushed tomatoes
- 1 large garlic clove, minced
- 3/4 tsp sea salt, or to taste
- 1 medium turnip, peeled, cut into 1/2-inch cubes (1 3/4 cups)
- 1 cup frozen peas, thawed
- 1/2 cup packed, chopped fresh herb mixture, such as flat-leaf parsley, mint, and basil (divided use)

DIRECTIONS

1. In a large bowl or sealable plastic bag, toss the lamb cubes with flour.

2. Heat the oil in a large nonstick pan over medium heat. Add the lamb and onions and cook, stirring frequently, for 10 minutes or until the lamb cubes are brown on all sides and the onions are lightly caramelized.

3. Place the cooked lamb and onions in a large saucepan over high heat. Add the water, tomatoes, garlic, and salt. Bring to a boil, then reduce heat to low, cover, and simmer for 10 minutes.

4. Add the turnips, cover, and simmer 40 minutes or until the turnips are just cooked through. Add the peas and half the herbs, cover, and simmer 5 minutes. Sprinkle with remaining herbs to serve.

Exchanges: 1 1/2 carbohydrate, 2 lean meat; 230 calories, 69 calories from fat, 8 g total fat, 2 g saturated fat, 40 mg cholesterol, 595 mg sodium, 23 g total carbohydrate, 6 g dietary fiber, 5 g sugars, 17 g protein.

FRESH FACT

If you've never had turnips or think you don't like them, this stew recipe is one of the most delicious ways to begin enjoying this cruciferous veggie. You'll find this white vegetable with purple-tinged skin available in the fall and winter—the ideal seasons for stew.

CHICKEN TORTILLA SOUP WITH CALIFORNIA AVOCADO

Serves 4/serving size: 1 1/4 cups

This muy delicioso soup has some of your favorite things—like avocado, tortilla chips, and chicken—all in one tantalizing dish. It may quickly become a family favorite.

- 3 cups natural fat-free chicken broth
- 1 2/3 cups canned organic crushed tomatoes
- 1 small jalapeño pepper with seeds, minced
- 2 large garlic cloves, minced
- 1 1/2 cups bite-size roasted chicken breast pieces (antibiotic free; 5 oz)
- 1/2 cup thinly sliced green onion
- 1/4 cup chopped fresh cilantro
- 2 Tbsp lime juice
- 1 1/2 oz unsalted blue corn tortilla chips, broken (not crushed; about 10 large or 15 medium chips)
- 1/2 Hass avocado, peeled and diced

DIRECTIONS

1. Bring the broth, tomatoes, jalapeño, and garlic to a boil in a large saucepan over high heat. Reduce the heat to medium and simmer 5 minutes.

2. Add the chicken and green onion; simmer 2 minutes. Remove from heat and stir in the cilantro and lime juice. Top with tortilla chips and avocado to serve.

Exchanges: 1/2 starch, 2 vegetable, 2 lean meat, 1/2 fat; 210 calories, 68 calories from fat, 8 g total fat, 1 g saturated fat, 30 mg cholesterol, 450 mg sodium, 19 g total carbohydrate, 5 g dietary fiber, 1 g sugars, 18 g protein.

FOOD FLAIR

Instead of tortilla chips, top this soup with crispy baked tortilla strips. Slice corn tortillas into thin strips and place on a baking sheet. Lightly coat strips with natural cooking spray. Bake in a 400°F oven until crisp and golden brown.

FAST FIX

Don't make chicken just for this soup—leftovers work great. Or pick up a rotisserie chicken from the market and use the chicken meat from one of the breasts. Serve the remaining roasted chicken as your entrée.

SIMPLE GAZPACHO

Serves 4/serving size: 1 cup

When tomatoes are fresh, seasonal, and fully ripened, they're ideal for making gazpacho . . . a perky and pretty soup that's served chilled. It's a taste bud treat for those who want fine food fast, too.

- 5 medium vine-ripened tomatoes, seeded and coarsely chopped (5 cups)
- 1 (5.5-oz) can spicy vegetable or tomato juice
- 1/2 cup thinly sliced green onion (divided use)
- 2 large garlic cloves, minced
- 2 Tbsp lime juice
- 1 1/2 tsp extra virgin olive oil
- 1/4 tsp freshly ground black pepper, or to taste

DIRECTIONS

1. Puree the tomatoes, vegetable juice, 1/4 cup green onion, garlic, lime juice, and oil in a blender on low speed until just combined. (If your blender has less than a 5-cup capacity, puree in two batches.)

2. Add pepper to taste. Serve chilled, topped with the remaining green onion.

Exchanges: 2 vegetable, 1/2 fat; 70 calories, 19 calories from fat, 2 g total fat, 0 g saturated fat, 0 mg cholesterol, 135 mg sodium, 11 g total carbohydrate, 3 g dietary fiber, 6 g sugars, 2 g protein.

FRESH FACT

What makes tomatoes so tasty when they're fully ripened? One reason is called umami—one of the five basic tastes (the others are sweet, salty, sour, and bitter). It provides a taste that many call "savory." Some foods naturally high in umami are mushrooms, parmesan cheese, soy sauce, balsamic vinegar, wine, and, yes, tomatoes. When these foods are aged—and when tomatoes are fully ripened, naturally processed into a tomato product, or cooked—the umami is enhanced.

MORE THAN FOUR?

This vibrant gazpacho is a party-friendly soup. It's tasty and not so typical. Plus, it's good cool or at room temperature, so there's no need to worry about proper timing. Serve this like a punch at the dining table for more "wow" factor.

TWO-IN-A-BOWL FRUIT SOUP

Serves 3/serving size: 1 cup

*Need a soup that'll impress your guests?
Look no further—this fabulously fruity soup is it.
You'll impress yourself, too.*

- 2 cups cubed honeydew melon
- 1/4 cup pear nectar
- 4 tsp fresh lime juice (divided use)
- 2 cups cubed cantaloupe
- 1/4 cup apricot nectar
- 4 sprigs fresh mint

1. Puree the honeydew, pear nectar, and 2 tsp lime juice in a blender until smooth. Pour into a small pitcher or large liquid measuring cup.

2. Puree the cantaloupe, apricot nectar, and remaining lime juice in the blender until smooth.

3. At same time and same rate, pour each of the soups into opposite sides of 3 small bowls, about 1/2 cup of each per bowl. Garnish with mint.

FOOD FLAIR

Get ambitious with this soup. Go for three-in-a-bowl by adding watermelon puree— 2 cups watermelon cubes, 1/4 cup guava or pear nectar, and 2 tsp lime juice. You'll then need another hand so you can pour all three soups into each bowl at once.

Exchanges: 1 1/2 fruit; 90 calories, 0 calories from fat, 0 g total fat, 0 g saturated fat, 0 mg cholesterol, 35 mg sodium, 23 g total carbohydrate, 2 g dietary fiber, 15 g sugars, 1 g protein.

BETWEEN
THE BREAD

AUTUMN ROASTED TURKEY WRAP WITH PUMPKIN PUREE AND CRANBERRY SAUCE

Serves 4/serving size: 1 wrap

Here's a way to experience the taste of Thanksgiving any time of the year—and without the tempting indulgences that go with it. This no-cook wrap has all the best of the holiday feast in one nutrient-rich package.

- 1 cup canned or fresh no-salt-added pumpkin puree
- 1/2 cup whole cranberry sauce
- 4 (8-inch) whole wheat or regular flour tortillas, lightly warmed
- 1 cup finely shredded romaine lettuce
- 1/4 cup minced fresh chives
- 8 large fresh sage leaves, thinly sliced
- 8 oz sliced natural low-sodium oven-roasted turkey deli meat

DIRECTIONS

1. Spread the pumpkin and cranberry sauce over the entire surface of each tortilla. Sprinkle each tortilla with lettuce, chives, and sage.

2. Top with turkey and roll up each filled tortilla. Secure closed with toothpicks, if needed. Slice in half diagonally to serve.

FRESH FACT

Like sweet potatoes and carrots, pumpkin is packed with beta-carotene. It's not necessary to use fresh roasted pumpkin. And it's not practical or possible to do so year-round. The canned variety is ideal —stock up on extra cans at the holidays so you can enjoy this Thanksgiving-inspired wrap any time.

Exchanges: 2 starch, 1 carbohydrate, 1 lean meat; 190 calories, 6 calories from fat, 1 g total fat, 0 g saturated fat, 25 mg cholesterol, 530 mg sodium, 38 g total carbohydrate, 4 g dietary fiber, 11 g sugars, 14 g protein.

RANCHER ROAST BEEF BUN

Serves 4/serving size: 1 sandwich

Go beyond mustard or mayonnaise as a sandwich spread. Here, Ranch dressing is the tangy condiment of choice. And there's no need to go light or fat-free with it. Just go lean on the other ingredients. Even roast beef is considered lean!

- 4 (2-oz) whole wheat buns, halved
- 2 Tbsp natural Ranch dressing
- 2 Tbsp finely crumbled blue cheese
- 4 large, thin slices Vidalia, Maui, or other sweet onion
- 1 1/2 cups organic baby arugula or torn regular arugula
- 6 oz thinly sliced lean deli roast beef (antibiotic free)
- 4 large, thin slices vine-ripened or beefsteak tomato
- 1/4 tsp freshly ground black pepper, or to taste

DIRECTIONS

1. On the bottom half of each bun, thinly spread the dressing, then sprinkle with blue cheese. Arrange the onion, arugula, roast beef, and tomato on top. Add pepper to taste.

2. Place the bun tops on the sandwiches and secure each with a frilly toothpick, if desired.

Exchanges: 2 starch, 2 lean meat, 1/2 fat; 280 calories, 81 calories from fat, 9 g total fat, 2 g saturated fat, 30 mg cholesterol, 380 mg sodium, 32 g total carbohydrate, 5 g dietary fiber, 6 g sugars, 19 g protein.

FRESH FACT

Some of the leanest cuts of beef include bottom round roast or steak, 95% lean ground beef, eye of round roast or steak, sirloin tip side steak, chuck shoulder pot roast, and round tip roast or steak.

MORE THAN FOUR?

Double or triple this recipe as needed. Make in advance, minus the dressing and tomato slices. Wrap and refrigerate. Just before serving, add tomato and spread the dressing on the top half of each bun. Easier yet, serve the dressing on the side.

BEER-BREWED SLOPPY JOES

Serves 4/serving size: 1 sandwich

*Cooking with beer is fun! And beer has some health benefits—
when consumed in moderation. Though alcohol generally burns
off during the cooking process, the rich flavor and nutritional
value remain. Best of all, you can serve this high-flavor food to
everyone. Shhh ... don't give away your trade secret.*

- 2 tsp extra virgin olive oil
- 2 cups chopped Vidalia, Maui, or other sweet onion
- 1 large jalapeño pepper with or without seeds, diced
- 1 1/2 cups diced green bell pepper
- 14 oz lean ground beef sirloin (antibiotic free)
- 1/2 cup lite beer
- 3 Tbsp organic ketchup
- 2 Tbsp organic tomato paste
- 1/2 tsp garlic salt, or to taste
- 4 whole grain hamburger buns, lightly toasted

DIRECTIONS

1. Heat the oil in a large nonstick skillet over medium heat. Add the onion, jalapeño, and bell pepper and cook, stirring, for 5 minutes.

2. Add the beef and cook, stirring occasionally, for 5 minutes or until the meat is cooked through.

3. Add the beer, ketchup, tomato paste, and garlic salt. Cook and stir for 5 minutes or until the mixture is thick and no liquid remains.

4. Spoon about 1 cup of the Sloppy Joe mixture into each bun and serve immediately.

Exchanges: 2 starch, 1 vegetable, 2 lean meat, 1/2 fat; 330 calories, 83 calories from fat, 9 g total fat, 2 g saturated fat, 45 mg cholesterol, 560 mg sodium, 36 g total carbohydrate, 6 g dietary fiber, 11 g sugars, 27 g protein.

FRESH FACT

It's up to you and your taste buds how spicy you want to make your Sloppy Joes. Since much of the heat is in the jalapeño seeds, here's a simple guide to determine how many of them to use: all the seeds = very hot; half the seeds = medium hot; no seeds = mild.

FOOD FLAIR

Add 1/4 tsp (or more) ground cinnamon to the Sloppy Joe mixture for a Greek flavor flair. Serve in whole wheat pita pockets. For Sloppy Joe Molé, add 1/4 tsp ground cinnamon plus 1/4 tsp natural unsweetened cocoa powder. Enjoy wrapped in a tortilla or serve like a stew along with baked corn tortilla chips.

FRESH TARRAGON CHICKEN SALAD WITH ALMONDS ON MARBLE RYE

Serves 4/serving size: 1 sandwich

There are many culinary techniques to get the most flavor from healthier foods. Here's one: prepare this salad a day before you want to serve it. Allowing the flavors to marry overnight makes this recipe extra lovable.

- 1 pound boneless, skinless chicken breast (antibiotic free), roasted or poached and cubed (2 1/2 cups)
- 1/2 cup thinly sliced celery (slice on diagonal)
- 1/4 cup minced Vidalia, Maui, or other sweet onion
- 3 Tbsp mayonnaise
- 3 Tbsp fat-free plain yogurt
- 1 Tbsp tarragon or white wine vinegar
- 1 Tbsp finely chopped fresh tarragon
- 1/2 tsp sea salt, or to taste
- 2 Tbsp sliced almonds, pan-toasted
- 8 (1-oz) slices marble rye bread

DIRECTIONS

1. In a large bowl, gently combine the chicken, celery, onion, mayonnaise, yogurt, vinegar, tarragon, and salt. Refrigerate until ready to serve.

2. Stir in the almonds just before serving. Serve about 3/4 cup chicken salad per sandwich. Slice each in half diagonally, if desired.

Exchanges: 2 starch, 1/2 fat; 350 calories, 120 calories from fat, 13 g total fat, 2 g saturated fat, 65 mg cholesterol, 540 mg sodium, 26 g total carbohydrate, 8 g dietary fiber, 1 g sugars, 29 g protein.

FRESH FACT

If you're roasting the chicken, cube it first and marinate the cubes in yogurt or buttermilk for 1 hour before cooking. It'll add extra tenderness and tanginess.

FOOD FLAIR

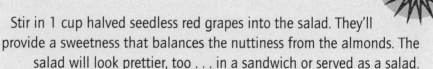

Stir in 1 cup halved seedless red grapes into the salad. They'll provide a sweetness that balances the nuttiness from the almonds. The salad will look prettier, too . . . in a sandwich or served as a salad.

FAST FIX

Buy a rotisserie chicken from the grocery store to use in this recipe. Remove the skin and shred the meat off the bone with your fingers. Use both the white and dark meat, if you choose. Though not as lean as the white, dark meat is still a healthful choice.

MORE THAN FOUR?

This chicken salad makes a lovely party food, especially when turned into a finger food. Place the chicken salad into a food processor and grind until smooth. Serve on small pieces of fresh or toasted rye bread. Garnish each with a fresh tarragon leaf or red grape half.

ROASTED RED BELL PEPPER, ARUGULA, AND GOAT CHEESE PUMPERNICKEL PANINI

Serves 4/serving size: 1 sandwich

The panini is the new sandwich. It takes just 5 more minutes to prepare than a regular sandwich, but it's so much more interesting. If you don't already have one, you may want to invest in an electric panini grill or other sandwich maker. It'll turn most of your healthy, humdrum sandwiches into happening ones.

- 1 1/3 oz soft goat cheese
- 3 Tbsp organic low-fat cottage cheese
- 2 tsp fresh lemon juice
- 1 large garlic clove, minced
- 1/2 tsp freshly ground black pepper, or to taste
- 8 (1-oz) slices pumpernickel or rye bread
- 1 (16-oz) jar roasted organic red bell peppers, well drained and cut into 12–16 pieces
- 16 large arugula leaves
- 12 large fresh basil leaves

DIRECTIONS

1. In a small bowl, stir the goat cheese, cottage cheese, lemon juice, garlic, and black pepper together until well combined.

2. Thinly spread the goat cheese mixture evenly on the top of each bread slice. Layer red pepper on top of 4 bread slices and top with the other slices.

3. Place each sandwich on a preheated panini grill over medium heat. Lightly place the lid on the sandwiches. Grill 5 minutes or

until toasted. Cook in batches, if necessary. Alternatively, pan-toast sandwiches in a preheated nonstick skillet over medium heat for 3 to 4 minutes per side, or until toasted.

4. Immediately fill each panini with arugula and basil. Slice each in half diagonally to serve.

Exchanges: 2 starch, 1/2 fat; 190 calories, 34 calories from fat, 4 g total fat, 1 g saturated fat, 5 mg cholesterol, 400 mg sodium, 29 g total carbohydrate, 9 g dietary fiber, 3 g sugars, 9 g protein.

FAST FIX

Make the goat cheese mixture in advance. Cover and refrigerate up to 3 days before you prepare the panini.

FOOD FLAIR

Add 1/2 Hass avocado, thinly sliced, to each panini sandwich after grilling. If you use avocado, stir 1 Tbsp instead of 2 tsp lemon juice into the goat cheese mixture. The panini will seem extra decadent.

BODACIOUS "STEAK" BURGER

Serves 4/serving size: 1 burger

Enjoying a lean hamburger doesn't have to mean switching to turkey burgers. Just choose a lean ground beef, like sirloin. And here's another trade secret: if you're worried your burgers will be too dry without the fat, just add some cottage cheese! Your burgers will be bodaciously moist.

- 1 lb lean ground beef sirloin (antibiotic free)
- 1/4 cup organic low-fat cottage cheese
- 1 Tbsp steak sauce
- 1 large garlic clove, minced
- 1/4 tsp sea salt, or to taste
- 1/4 tsp freshly ground black pepper, or to taste
- 4 whole wheat hamburger buns, toasted
- 4 large thin slices red onion
- 1 cup organic baby arugula

DIRECTIONS

1. Preheat the grill over medium-high heat. In a large bowl, gently combine the beef, cottage cheese, steak sauce, garlic, salt, and pepper with your hands. Lightly form the mixture into 4 even patties, about 1/3 inch thick.

2. Cook burgers for 4 to 5 minutes per side or until cooked at least to medium doneness.

3. Remove the burgers to a plate, cover with foil, and let rest for 5 minutes. Serve on buns with onion and arugula. Serve condiments on the side, if desired.

Exchanges: 1 1/2 starch, 3 lean meat; 290 calories, 67 calories from fat, 7 g total fat, 2 g saturated fat, 55 mg cholesterol, 490 mg sodium, 25 g total carbohydrate, 4 g dietary fiber, 5 g sugars, 30 g protein.

FRESH FACT

Though steaks can be cooked medium rare, it's important that ground beef be cooked a little longer, to at least medium doneness. How do you know when it's cooked properly? Use a meat thermometer. To help prevent food-borne illness, these ground sirloin burgers should reach an internal temperature of at least 160°F.

FAST FIX

Cook burgers inside instead of outdoors. Place a nonstick sauté pan over medium-high heat. Cook burgers (in batches, if necessary) for 3 minutes per side, or until at least medium doneness. You'll probably need to use the kitchen fan for this preparation. Or preheat broiler. Cook burgers on broiler pan under the broiler for 2 minutes per side, or until at least medium doneness.

MOROCCAN TURKEY BURGER PITA WITH YOGURT–CUMIN DRESSING

Serves 4/serving size: 1 burger

These burgers are filled with exotic flavors from olives, currants, and cinnamon. They also provide diabetes-friendly fiber—from oats. That makes these burgers good-tasting and good for you, too.

- 1 (5.3-oz) container fat-free Greek yogurt or 1/2 cup yogurt cheese (see recipe, page 63)
- 1/4 cup organic ketchup
- 1/4 tsp ground cumin
- 1 lb 93% lean ground turkey (antibiotic free)
- 1/3 cup grated Vidalia, Maui, or other sweet onion
- 6 pimento-stuffed green olives, minced
- 1 packet plain instant oatmeal (1/3 cup)
- 1/4 cup dried currants
- 1/4 tsp ground cinnamon
- 2 whole wheat pitas, halved
- 1 cup organic baby spinach (optional)

DIRECTIONS

1. In a small bowl, combine the yogurt, ketchup, and cumin.

2. In a medium bowl, combine the turkey, onion, olives, oatmeal, currants, and cinnamon with your hands. Make 4 oval patties, about 2/3 inch thick.

3. Place a large nonstick skillet over medium heat. Add the patties and cook for 5 minutes per side or until well done.

4. Stuff each pita half with a turkey patty, 2 1/2 Tbsp yogurt–cumin dressing, and spinach (if using).

Exchanges: 2 1/2 starch, 3 lean meat; 340 calories, 89 calories from fat, 10 g total fat, 2 g saturated fat, 65 mg cholesterol, 530 mg sodium, 35 g total carbohydrate, 4 g dietary fiber, 10 g sugars, 30 g protein.

FRESH FACT

Vidalia onions are seasonal in May and June. But if you're preparing this recipe from July through April, shop for other sweet onions, such as Maui, Oso Sweet, Walla Walla, and Rio Sweet. And since these onions are so sweet, mild, and crisp, they're wonderful raw, thinly sliced, and added to these burgers, too.

PAN-GRILLED VEGGIE CIABATTA WITH BALSAMIC— BASIL TOFUNNAISE

Serves 4/serving size: 1 sandwich

If you don't think you're a fan of tofu, you'll soon become one after a taste of the tofunnaise in this sandwich. (And you'll be a bigger fan if you already like tofu.) The tofunnaise is creamy like mayonnaise, but bursting with flavor from the balsamic vinegar, garlic, and basil. It's a perfect complement here to the avocado and veggies.

- 4 oz soft silken tofu, drained (1/2 cup)
- 2 Tbsp aged balsamic vinegar
- 1 large garlic clove
- 8 large fresh basil leaves
- 1 medium zucchini, sliced vertically into 4 slices
- 1 medium red bell pepper, cut into 8 pieces
- 1 (10-oz) loaf ciabatta bread, cut in half horizontally
- 1 Hass avocado, peeled and sliced
- 1/4 tsp sea salt, or to taste
- 1/4 cup thinly sliced red onion

DIRECTIONS

1. Puree the tofu, vinegar, garlic, and basil in a blender until smooth. Refrigerate the tofunnaise until ready to use.

2. Heat a nonstick grill pan over medium-high heat. Lightly coat the zucchini and bell pepper slices with natural cooking spray. Cook the vegetables 4 minutes per side or until done as desired.

FAST FIX

Store the tofunnaise tightly covered in the refrigerator up to 3 days. For a fiber boost, use 8 thin slices of whole wheat or pumpernickel bread instead of the ciabatta bread.

FOOD FLAIR

For a scrumptious taste of the great outdoors,
heat the grill over medium-high heat. Grill the
vegetables 4 to 5 minutes per side or until lightly
charred and cooked through, turning only as needed.

3. Spread the tofunnaise evenly on both cut surfaces of the bread. Top one half with zucchini, pepper, avocado, salt, and onion. Top with the other bread loaf half and skewer with long toothpicks or small bamboo skewers. Cut into 4 pieces to serve.

Exchanges: 2 1/2 starch, 1 vegetable, 1 1/2 fat; 300 calories, 85 calories from fat, 9 g total fat, 2 g saturated fat, 0 mg cholesterol, 430 mg sodium, 46 g total carbohydrate, 6 g dietary fiber, 5 g sugars, 9 g protein.

! FRESH FACT

Look for a ciabatta bread loaf that's long and flat, not big and round. If you find your loaf of bread too "bready," simply remove some of the inside bread by pinching it out with your fingers. Use that bread for another recipe—or for the birds.

SWEET POTATO BURRITO SPIRALS WITH BELL PEPPER— AVOCADO "CRÈME" SAUCE

Serves 4/serving size: 3 spirals

Better than any ordinary burrito, this delicious translation is like art on the plate—and the palate.

- 1 cup canned organic vegetarian refried beans
- 3 large (10-inch) whole wheat or regular flour tortillas, warmed
- 1 1/2 cups diced cooked or canned sweet potatoes, drained
- 1 Hass avocado, peeled and thinly sliced (divided use)
- 2/3 cup thinly sliced green onion (green part only)
- 1 1/2 cups finely shredded romaine lettuce
- 1/4 cup chopped fresh cilantro
- 1 1/2 cups chopped red bell pepper
- 1 small jalapeño pepper with seeds, sliced
- 2 Tbsp thinly sliced green onion (white part only)
- 2 Tbsp lime juice

DIRECTIONS

1. Spread the beans over the entire surface of each tortilla. Top with sweet potatoes, half the avocado, green part of the green onion, lettuce, and cilantro.

2. As tightly as possible, roll each filled tortilla. Slice diagonally with a bread knife into 4 pieces each.

3. Place a medium nonstick skillet over medium-high heat. Sauté the bell pepper, jalapeño, white part of the green onion, and lime juice for 5 minutes or until the peppers are softened. Place the pepper

mixture (including any browned bits) and the remaining avocado into a blender. Pulse until combined, then puree for 1 minute on high speed. If necessary, add up to 2 Tbsp cold water for proper blending.

4. Spoon about 1/3 cup of the warm (or room temperature) bell pepper sauce onto each of 4 plates. Arrange 3 burrito spirals, cut side up, on each sauce portion.

Exchanges: 3 1/2 starch, 1 vegetable, 1 fat; 340 calories, 82 calories from fat, 9 g total fat, 2 g saturated fat, 0 mg cholesterol, 380 mg sodium, 59 g total carbohydrate, 11 g dietary fiber, 10 g sugars, 12 g protein.

FAST FIX

Make the burritos in advance. Wrap each tightly in plastic wrap and chill. When you're ready to serve, slice the burritos in the wrap with a bread knife. Remove the wrap before arranging them on a plate. This will keep the spirals neatly in shape.

UNO, DOS, TRES BEAN BURRITO

Serves 4/serving size: 1 burrito

Bite for bite it doesn't get much more nutritious than this. Best of all, it doesn't get much tastier than this. Olé!

- 1 tsp canola or peanut oil
- 2 cups thinly sliced red onion
- 1/2 cup organic canned black beans, drained
- 1/2 cup organic canned small white or white cannellini beans, drained
- 1/2 cup organic canned pinto or Roman beans, drained
- 1/2 cup organic hot or medium chunky salsa
- 1/4 cup chopped fresh cilantro
- 4 (10-inch) whole wheat or regular flour tortillas, warmed
- 1/3 cup shredded Monterey Jack cheese
- 2 cups mesclun or other mixed baby greens

DIRECTIONS

1. Heat the oil in a large nonstick skillet over medium-high heat. Sauté the onion 5 minutes or until lightly caramelized. Add the beans and sauté 2 minutes. Stir in the salsa and cilantro and remove the skillet from the heat.

2. Spoon about 1/2 cup bean mixture onto each tortilla. Add the cheese and greens. Tightly roll each tortilla, tucking in the sides. Serve immediately, seam side down.

Exchanges: 2 1/2 starch, 1 vegetable, 1/2 fat; 240 calories, 43 calories from fat, 5 g total fat, 2 g saturated fat, 10 mg cholesterol, 500 mg sodium, 44 g total carbohydrate, 8 g dietary fiber, 8 g sugars, 12 g protein.

FOOD FLAIR

Slice the burritos in half diagonally for a pretty presentation. Also, use a different variety of beans each time you make these. See how many flavorful combinations you can come up with.

FAST FIX

This burrito is already a quick fix. But if you feel the need for more speed, serve with one type of bean instead of three. After it's drained, one (15-oz) can of beans is about 1 1/2 cups— the exact amount you need for this recipe.

MORE THAN FOUR?

Leave out the greens when making the burritos in advance or if you're planning to serve them later. Just reheat in the microwave and add the greens just before serving—or serve them on the side as a salad.

TAKE-AWAY THAI CHICKEN TORTILLA ROLL-UP

Serves 4/serving size: 1 roll-up

Consider this chicken roll-up as healthful, homemade fast food. It's so easy to make, even kids can get into the act.

- 1/4 cup Thai peanut satay sauce
- 4 (10-inch) whole wheat or regular flour tortillas
- 2 1/2 cups bite-size roasted chicken breast pieces (antibiotic free), chilled (12 oz)
- 2 cups fresh mung bean sprouts
- 3/4 cup thinly sliced green onion
- 2 Tbsp finely chopped fresh cilantro

DIRECTIONS

1. Spread the peanut sauce over the entire surface of each tortilla. Top with chicken, sprouts, green onion, and cilantro.

2. Roll each tortilla and secure closed with a decorative toothpick, if necessary.

Exchanges: 2 1/2 starch, 3 lean meat; 370 calories, 80 calories from fat, 9 g total fat, 2 g saturated fat, 70 mg cholesterol, 430 mg sodium, 39 g total carbohydrate, 4 g dietary fiber, 3 g sugars, 38 g protein.

FAST FIX

Use rotisserie chicken from the grocery store. Remove the skin from the breast and shred the meat off the bone with your fingers. Or, make extra chicken when you plan it as an entrée. Freeze chicken leftovers in airtight plastic wrap or a plastic freezer bag; thaw overnight in the refrigerator to use in the roll-ups.

FOOD FLAIR

Try with 1 1/3 cups coleslaw mix (shredded cabbage with carrots) instead of the sprouts for a change of taste.

AFTERNOON DELIGHT TUNA SALAD SANDWICH

Serves 4/serving size: 1 sandwich

This sandwich is definitely delightful in the afternoon. But don't let that stop you from enjoying it any time of the day. The secret is having just enough real mayo to marry all ingredients together.

- 1 (7-oz) can water-packed solid tuna, drained and separated into chunks
- 1 1/4 cups thinly sliced celery (slice on diagonal)
- 8 cherry tomatoes, thinly sliced
- 1/4 cup finely diced Vidalia, Maui, or other sweet onion
- 3 Tbsp chopped fresh Italian parsley
- 3 Tbsp chopped fresh cilantro
- 3 Tbsp lemon juice
- 2 Tbsp mayonnaise
- 1 Tbsp spicy Dijon mustard
- 8 (1-oz) slices whole grain bread

DIRECTIONS

1. In a medium bowl, combine the tuna, celery, tomatoes, onion, parsley, cilantro, lemon juice, mayonnaise, and mustard.

2. Spread the mixture on top of 4 slices of bread. Top with remaining bread slices and cut in half diagonally.

Exchanges: 2 starch, 1 lean meat, 1 fat; 260 calories, 73 calories from fat, 8 g total fat, 1 g saturated fat, 15 mg cholesterol, 520 mg sodium, 30 g total carbohydrate, 5 g dietary fiber, 8 g sugars, 16 g protein.

FRESH FACT

Italian, or flat-leaf, parsley is often confused with cilantro, so don't be fooled. The leaf tips of flat-leaf parsley are somewhat pointed, while cilantro's are more rounded and delicate. When in doubt, rub a leaf of each in your fingers and take a whiff. The cilantro will be more pungent.

FOOD FLAIR

Use this recipe as a simple starting point for your own ideas, then change ingredients to suit yourself. Like it spicier? Add more mustard. Like more Mexican than Italian flavors? Increase the cilantro and decrease the parsley.

ANCHO CHILI LIME-DRESSED GREENS ON FLATBREAD WITH SMOKED TURKEY

Serves 4/serving size: 1 sandwich

The ancho chili is the sweetest of the dried chilis. So its powder adds pleasant, yet pungent taste to this turkey sandwich without overpowering the rest of the ingredients. Savor it as a salad and sandwich all in one.

- 2 Tbsp lime juice
- 1 Tbsp mayonnaise
- 2 tsp acacia or other mild floral honey
- 1/2 tsp ancho or other chili powder
- 4 cups mesclun or other mixed baby greens
- 2 Tbsp finely chopped fresh cilantro
- 4 oz thinly sliced natural low-sodium smoked turkey deli meat
- 4 (8-inch) pocketless whole grain Middle Eastern flatbread

DIRECTIONS

1. In a medium bowl, whisk the lime juice, mayonnaise, honey, and chili powder.

2. Add the greens and cilantro and toss until well coated.

3. Divide the turkey among the flatbread and top with dressed greens. Fold to eat.

Exchanges: 2 1/2 starch, 1 lean meat, 1/2 fat; 280 calories, 67 calories from fat, 7 g total fat, 1 g saturated fat, 15 mg cholesterol, 590 mg sodium, 41 g total carbohydrate, 5 g dietary fiber, 6 g sugars, 13 g protein.

FRESH FACT

In its fresh form, the ancho chili is called poblano. It's the chili used to make chili rellenos—cheese-stuffed peppers.

FOOD FLAIR

Add an Indian touch by using toasted naan (Indian flatbread). Then serve the recipe pizza-style, rather than as a sandwich. For more Southwestern appeal, add all ingredients to a whole-wheat flour tortilla. Roll up burrito-style.

HORSERADISH PORK TENDERLOIN ON NAAN WITH ARUGULA

Serves 4/serving size: 1 sandwich

This "other white meat" is extremely lean. Make lean become lovable by pairing this pork with high-flavored horseradish, rosemary, Dijon mustard, and arugula. It's a memorable mouthful.

- 8 oz lean pork tenderloin, trimmed of fat (antibiotic free)
- 2 Tbsp prepared horseradish (divided use)
- 2 large garlic cloves, minced
- 1 tsp minced fresh rosemary
- 1/8 tsp sea salt, or to taste
- 1/4 tsp freshly ground black pepper, or to taste
- 2 Tbsp Dijon mustard
- 1 Tbsp mayonnaise
- 4 (8-inch) naan (Indian flatbread)
- 2 cups organic baby arugula or chopped regular arugula

DIRECTIONS

1. Preheat the oven to 450°F. Place the pork tenderloin on a nonstick baking pan.

2. In small bowl, stir together 1 Tbsp horseradish, garlic, rosemary, salt, and pepper. Rub and press mixture with your fingers over the entire surface of the pork.

3. Roast in the oven for 20 minutes or until cooked through and just slightly pink in the center. Remove from the oven and let stand for at least 5 minutes, then thinly slice the pork.

4. In a small bowl, stir together the mustard, mayonnaise, and remaining horseradish and spread the mixture on the flatbread. Arrange the arugula and pork on the flatbread. Fold and enjoy.

Exchanges: 2 1/2 starch, 2 lean meat; 300 calories, 79 calories from fat, 9 g total fat, 2 g saturated fat, 35 mg cholesterol, 570 mg sodium, 37 g total carbohydrate, 4 g dietary fiber, 3 g sugars, 19 g protein.

FRESH FACT

Arugula is a leafy green with a peppery kick that adds so much enjoyment to sandwiches, salads, and pastas. Look for it year-round, but especially late in the summer. It might also be labeled as rocket, rocket salad, roquette, rucola, or gharghir, depending on where you buy it.

FOOD FLAIR

Since naan is nearly always found as a white bread, give whole grain varieties of pita, pocketless Middle Eastern flatbread, lavash (a soft, thin flatbread), or tortillas a try. Not only will these boost your whole grain intake, they'll let you enjoy this sandwich in various ways. Just stuff the pita or fill and roll the flatbread, lavash, or tortilla.

STUFFED LEMONY HUMMUS PITA

Serves 4/serving size: 1 sandwich

Hummus is best known and usually enjoyed as a velvety Middle Eastern dip. But it's equally enticing when served in a sandwich. And, any way it's eaten, it's still a fantastic fiber source for everyone.

- 1 (15-oz) can organic chickpeas (garbanzo beans), drained
- 2 large garlic cloves
- 3 Tbsp tahini (sesame paste)

- 1/4 cup lemon juice
- 2 Tbsp water
- 1/4 tsp sea salt, or to taste
- 2 whole wheat pitas, halved

- 1 1/3 cups thinly sliced English (hothouse) cucumber with skin
- 8 cherry tomatoes, thinly sliced
- 1/3 cup thinly sliced green onion

DIRECTIONS

1. Puree the chickpeas, garlic, tahini, lemon juice, water, and salt in a blender until smooth, adding more water by tablespoonfuls only if necessary.

2. Spread about 1/3 cup hummus into each of the pita halves. Stuff with the cucumber, tomatoes, and green onion.

Exchanges: 2 1/2 starch, 1 fat; 240 calories, 70 calories from fat, 8 g total fat, 1 g saturated fat, 0 mg cholesterol, 390 mg sodium, 35 g total carbohydrate, 8 g dietary fiber, 5 g sugars, 10 g protein.

FOOD FLAIR

Try the Jalapeño-Peanut Hummus (see recipe, page 59) instead of this version for a little extra kick.

FRESH FACT

If you add a little more water when blending the hummus, you can serve it as a dip with pita wedges and veggies on the side, rather than as a sandwich filling.

ELEGANT & EASY ENTRÉES

TRUFFLED BEEF TENDERLOIN PIZZETTE

Serves 4/serving size: 1 piece

This thin and crispy pizza tastes like a million bucks! The tenderloin and truffle oil make it an indulgent treat. And at less than 200 calories a serving, this balanced bite will be a popular pick. Go ahead, indulge!

- 2 (2-oz) whole wheat or regular lavash flatbreads
- 6 oz lean beef tenderloin (antibiotic free), cut into 24 thin, bite-size pieces
- 1/3 cup shredded part-skim mozzarella cheese
- 1/4 cup very thinly sliced red onion
- 1/4 tsp garlic salt
- 1/4 tsp freshly ground black pepper, or to taste
- 2 tsp white truffle oil
- 1/4 cup chopped fresh flat-leaf parsley

DIRECTIONS

1. Preheat the broiler. Place the flatbreads on a large baking sheet and broil for 1 minute or until lightly toasted.

2. Turn flatbreads over on baking sheet, broiled side down. Top the entire surface of each with half the beef, cheese, and onion. Sprinkle with garlic salt and pepper. Broil for 1 minute or until flatbreads are lightly toasted and beef is browned. Remove from the oven.

3. Reduce heat to 450°F. When the oven is ready, bake on the middle rack for 5 minutes or until beef is done as desired. Remove from the oven and immediately drizzle with oil and sprinkle with parsley. Cut each pizzette in half and serve immediately.

Exchanges: 1 starch, 1 lean meat, 1 fat; 170 calories, 60 calories from fat, 7 g total fat, 2 g saturated fat, 30 mg cholesterol, 280 mg sodium, 17 g total carbohydrate, 2 g dietary fiber, 2 g sugars, 14 g protein.

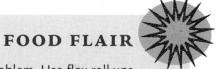

FOOD FLAIR

Can't find lavash flatbread? No problem. Use flax roll-ups or large whole wheat tortillas instead. Or for thick crust lovers, try pocketless whole wheat pita bread.

ASIAN SESAME SOBA NOODLE BOWL WITH BELL PEPPERS AND SNOW PEAS

Serves 4/serving size: 1 cup noodles plus veggies

Tired of regular ol' noodles? Then slurp up these soba noodles. Soba noodles add depth of flavor and Asian flair. Plus, they're made with buckwheat, a whole grain that might be helpful in the management of diabetes.

- 8 oz dry soba noodles
- 1/4 cup rice vinegar
- 1/3 cup thinly sliced green onion
- 2 Tbsp acacia or other mild floral honey

- 1 1/2 Tbsp naturally brewed reduced-sodium soy sauce
- 1 Tbsp grated fresh ginger root
- 1 1/2 tsp Asian garlic–chili sauce, or to taste
- 2 Tbsp toasted sesame oil

- 1 medium red bell pepper, thinly sliced (1 cup)
- 1 cup snow pea pods, ends trimmed, whole, or 1/2 cup thinly sliced lengthwise (several times)

DIRECTIONS

1. Cook the noodles according to package directions, omitting added oil and salt. Meanwhile, in a small bowl, whisk together the vinegar, green onion, honey, soy sauce, ginger root, and chili sauce.

2. Drain the noodles and place in a large bowl. Sprinkle with oil and toss to coat. Add the sauce and toss again. Chill in the refrigerator, stirring occasionally to prevent sticking.

3. Just before serving, stir in most of the peppers and snow peas, saving the rest for garnish. Serve at room temperature or chilled in a bowl with chopsticks.

Exchanges: 4 starch, 1/2 fat; 330 calories, 63 calories from fat, 7 g total fat, 1 g saturated fat, 0 mg cholesterol, 440 mg sodium, 59 g total carbohydrate, 4 g dietary fiber, 10 g sugars, 12 g protein.

FRESH FACT

Most bell peppers start their lives being green. So red bell peppers are actually ripened green bell peppers. And that ripening is what makes them taste sweet. They're available year-round, but at their peak in the summer.

FOOD FLAIR

To turn this entrée into a one-dish meal, make extra sauce to use as a marinade for flank steak or boneless, skinless chicken. Grill the marinated steak or chicken, thinly slice, and serve on top of the noodles. For added sesame flavor plus extra texture and eye appeal, sprinkle with toasted sesame seeds. And top with cilantro for a fresh finish.

FREE-RANGE GARLIC CHICKEN SCAMPI WITH ARUGULA

Serves 4/serving size: rounded 1 1/2 cups

So light, so satisfying, so simple, this meal-in-one pasta dish is so decidedly delicious that you won't realize it's nutritious. Try it with some freshly grated Parmigiana–Reggiano cheese for a jolt of pure pleasure.

- 14 oz free-range boneless, skinless chicken breast (antibiotic free), cut into large, thin, bite-size pieces
- 2 Tbsp extra virgin olive oil
- 4 large garlic cloves, minced
- 1 Tbsp thinly sliced green onion (white part only)
- 1/4 cup lemon juice
- 8 oz dry whole wheat linguine
- 1 tsp unsalted butter
- 1 bunch fresh arugula, torn into large pieces, or 1 (5-oz) package organic baby arugula
- 1/3 cup thinly sliced green onion (green part only)
- 3/4 tsp sea salt, or to taste
- 1/2 tsp freshly ground black pepper, or to taste

DIRECTIONS

1. Preheat the oven to 400°F. Place the chicken pieces, oil, garlic, white part of the green onion, and lemon juice in a deep-sided 9 × 13-inch baking pan. Stir to coat, then bake for 12 minutes or until the chicken is fully cooked.

2. Meanwhile, cook the linguine according to package directions, omitting added oil and salt. Drain the linguine, return to the pot, and toss with butter.

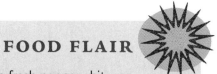

FOOD FLAIR

For more fresh peppery bite, go heavy on arugula: use two bunches instead of one. And before squeezing the lemon juice, grate its peel. Use this lemon zest as an additional flavorful ingredient along with an extra drizzle of olive oil before serving. It'll kick up the flavor a few notches. Then, for an interesting texture twist, serve topped with toasted pine nuts.

3. Stir the arugula and green onion into the chicken, then toss the chicken mixture with the linguine. Sprinkle with salt and pepper. Serve hot on a large platter.

Exchanges: 2 1/2 starch, 1 vegetable, 3 lean meat; 390 calories, 102 calories from fat, 11 g total fat, 2 g saturated fat, 55 mg cholesterol, 500 mg sodium, 45 g total carbohydrate, 8 g dietary fiber, 2 g sugars, 29 g protein.

FRESH FACT

Chicken can be labeled "free range" when the animals were given outdoor access. Interestingly, chickens choose not to roam far; they often stay close to their water and feed within their "houses." So, they may provide limited nutritional advantages to conventionally raised chickens. Though not all free-range chicken is organic, if the chicken is labeled "USDA Organic," it will be free range. Plus, the chickens at least get to experience some freedom. For you, it's basically personal preference which type of chicken you choose.

TEQUILA–LIME CHICKEN WITH SPINACH FETTUCCINE IN CREAMY JALAPEÑO SAUCE

Serves 4/serving size: 1 1/2 cups

Whether your past experience with tequila has been good, bad, or nonexistent, the experience you'll have while eating this tangy tequila pasta is all good. And don't worry about feeding this to kids; generally no alcohol remains after sautéing.

- 8 oz dry spinach or whole wheat fettuccine
- 1 Tbsp extra virgin olive oil
- 1 lb boneless, skinless chicken breast (antibiotic free), cut lengthwise into 16 thin pieces
- 2 cups thinly sliced red onion
- 1 large jalapeño pepper with seeds, finely chopped
- 1/2 cup tequila (see Fresh Fact)
- 1/4 cup lime juice (divided use)
- 1 1/2 tsp garlic salt (divided use)
- 1/4 cup freshly grated Parmigiana-Reggiano cheese
- 1/4 cup fat-free evaporated milk
- 1/4 cup chopped fresh cilantro

DIRECTIONS

1. Cook the fettuccine according to package directions, omitting added oil and salt. Drain the pasta, reserving 1/4 cup cooking liquid.

2. Meanwhile, heat the oil in an extra-large nonstick skillet over medium heat. Sauté the chicken, onion, and jalapeño for 10 minutes or until the chicken is done. Add the tequila and 2 Tbsp lime juice. Sauté for 5 minutes or until the liquid has evaporated, yet the mixture is still moist. Stir in 1/2 tsp garlic salt.

FOOD FLAIR

For beautiful balance and added nutrients, toss in 2 cups sliced
red or yellow bell pepper—or a pepper mixture—to this pasta recipe.
Sauté the peppers for 1 minute in the pan along with the chicken,
onion, and jalapeño just before adding the tequila. Serve in a colorful
bowl with additional grated cheese and lime wedges, if desired.

3. Add the pasta to the chicken mixture and toss, using long-handled
   tongs. Add the cheese, reserved cooking water, evaporated milk,
   remaining lime juice, and remaining garlic salt. Toss to combine
   well. Remove from heat once the liquid is absorbed, top with cilantro, and serve immediately.

Exchanges: 3 1/2 starch, 4 lean meat; 490 calories, 78 calories from fat, 9
g total fat, 2 g saturated fat, 70 mg cholesterol, 530 mg sodium, 50 g total
carbohydrate, 4 g dietary fiber, 5 g sugars, 34 g protein.

FRESH FACT

If you're unsure whether you'll like tequila in your food, try this recipe with 1/4
cup tequila and 1/4 cup natural chicken or vegetable broth. And, if you want to forgo the
tequila, use 1/3 cup broth and the juice of another lime.

JALAPEÑO WHOLE WHEAT LINGUINE PESTO WITH POACHED CHICKEN AND SUN-DRIED TOMATOES

Serves 4/serving size: 2 cups

Have your pesto and eat it, too. This linguine is tossed with a healthful, yet full-flavored, pesto sauce. Broth replaces part of the oil to keep calories in check.

- 8 oz dry whole wheat linguine
- 1 recipe Basil-Pine Nut Pesto (see Fresh Fact)
- 12 oz poached, grilled, or roasted boneless, skinless chicken breast (antibiotic free), thinly sliced (about 2 cups sliced; see Fresh Fact)
- 1 medium yellow, orange, or red bell pepper, thinly sliced (1 cup)
- 1 large jalapeño pepper with or without seeds, thinly sliced crosswise
- 10 dry-packed sun-dried tomato halves, thinly sliced (1/4 cup)
- 1/4 tsp sea salt, or to taste
- 2 Tbsp freshly grated Parmigiana-Reggiano cheese

DIRECTIONS

1. Cook the linguine in a large saucepot according to package directions, omitting added oil and salt, until just al dente. Drain the pasta, reserving 1/2 cup cooking liquid.

2. Place the saucepot over medium heat. Return the pasta to the pot with the reserved cooking liquid and toss with all ingredients except the cheese, using long-handled tongs. Continue to toss for 3 minutes or until the cooking liquid is absorbed. Sprinkle with cheese.

Exchanges: 3 starch, 4 lean meat; 440 calories, 105 calories from fat, 12 g total fat, 2 g saturated fat, 75 mg cholesterol, 580 mg sodium, 48 g total carbohydrate, 9 g dietary fiber, 5 g sugars, 38 g protein.

FRESH FACTS

Here's how to make Basil–Pine Nut Pesto. In a small food processor, puree 2 large peeled garlic cloves, 1 cup packed fresh basil leaves, 3 Tbsp natural vegetable or chicken broth, 2 Tbsp pine nuts, 1 Tbsp extra virgin olive oil, 1 Tbsp grated Parmigiana-Reggiano cheese, and 1/4 tsp sea salt. Make pesto ahead of time; it refrigerates or freezes well (makes about 1/2 cup).

To poach the chicken for this recipe, start with 1 lb raw chicken breast meat to yield 12 oz cooked. Place the chicken in a large saucepan with a handful of cubed carrots, onions, and celery. Cover with water. Add other flavorings, if desired, such as a splash of white wine vinegar or lemon juice, bay leaf, peppercorns, dried rosemary, and garlic. Bring to a boil, then skim off any foam that forms. Reduce the heat to low and partially cover. Gently simmer until the chicken is done. Remove the chicken to a cutting board and let rest at least 10 minutes before cutting. For best results, slice poached chicken when slightly cooled or completely chilled. Reserve some of the poaching liquid and drizzle it on the chicken slices to keep them moist.

FOOD FLAIR

Keep the skin on chicken while you grill or roast it, then remove the skin afterward. This helps keep the chicken meat moist during the cooking process.

Dry-packed sun-dried tomatoes often need to be hydrated. Simply soak them in simmering vegetable or tomato juice until they're the texture you like. Drain excess liquid once tomatoes are hydrated.

FAST FIXES

Use commercially prepared basil pesto. The downside: you can only use about 2 1/2 Tbsp of it (not 1/2 cup!) to stay within healthful recipe guidelines for diabetes.

Go ahead and cheat with this recipe and use a rotisserie chicken from the grocery store. Just remove the chicken from the bone and take the skin off the breast before slicing.

CREOLE-STYLE RED BEANS AND RICE

Serves 4/serving size: 1/2 cup beans over 1/3 cup rice

The soluble fiber-filled kidney beans in this entrée may help control blood glucose levels. But, don't think of the fiber when you eat this . . . think of the New Orleans-inspired taste. It tastes like the beans have been simmered for hours. And that's downright delicious.

- 1 Tbsp extra virgin olive oil
- 3 (1-oz) slices organic turkey bacon, chopped
- 1/2 cup chopped white onion
- 3 large garlic cloves, chopped
- 1 (15-oz) can organic kidney beans, drained
- 1/2 cup natural fat-free chicken or vegetable broth
- 1 large vine-ripened or beef-steak tomato, seeded and diced (1 1/3 cups)
- 1/2 tsp ground cayenne red pepper
- 1/4 tsp sea salt, or to taste
- 1 1/3 cups cooked brown basmati rice, warm

DIRECTIONS

1. Heat the oil in a large saucepan or deep skillet over medium heat. Add the bacon, onion, and garlic; sauté for 7 minutes or until the bacon is cooked and the onion is slightly caramelized.

2. Stir in the kidney beans, broth, tomato, red pepper, and salt. Cover and cook for 10 minutes, or until the flavors are blended and mixture is thick, stirring occasionally.

3. Ladle the bean mixture over the rice and serve.

Exchanges: 2 starch, 1 1/2 fat; 230 calories, 79 calories from fat, 9 g total fat, 2 g saturated fat, 20 mg cholesterol, 520 mg sodium, 29 g total carbohydrate, 5 g dietary fiber, 4 g sugars, 10 g protein.

FRESH FACT !

Fresh herbs can add fragrance and flavor along with antioxidants to a finished dish. For that antioxidant boost here, stir finely chopped fresh oregano or thyme leaves into the cooked beans or rice—or both.

FOOD FLAIR

Make your own salt-free Creole seasoning blend, and use 1 1/2 tsp in place of the 1/2 tsp cayenne red pepper in this recipe. Simple combine 2 Tbsp sweet paprika; 1 Tbsp each onion powder, garlic powder, and dried oregano; and 2 tsp each dried thyme leaves, celery seed, cayenne red pepper, and black pepper in a sealable plastic bag or container. Shake until well combined (makes about 1/2 cup).

FAST FIX

Prepare rice up to 2 days in advance and chill. It can be quickly reheated in the microwave. To make approximately 1 1/3 cups cooked brown basmati rice, simmer 1/2 cup rice with 1 cup water according to package directions, omitting added oil or salt. Want something faster? If you have 10 minutes, try a box of quick-cooking brown rice.

EYE OF ROUND STEAK WITH ORGANIC RED WINE REDUCTION SAUCE

Serves 4/serving size: 1 steak plus 2 Tbsp sauce

There's nothing quite like a succulent steak, especially when you can feel good about enjoying it. You can impress guests (and yourself) by serving grass-finished beef, a trendy but oh-so-healthful choice. Grass-finished beef is from animals that have been pasture-fed their entire lives.

- 2 tsp vegetable or canola oil
- 16 oz grass-finished beef eye of round (antibiotic free), trimmed of fat, cut into 4 steaks (1 inch thick)
- 1/2 tsp sea salt, or to taste (divided use)
- 1/2 tsp freshly ground black pepper, or to taste
- 1 tsp unsalted butter
- 1/3 cup sliced green onion
- 1 large garlic clove, minced
- 1 tsp minced fresh rosemary leaves
- 3/4 cup organic red wine
- 1/2 cup natural fat-free beef-flavored broth

DIRECTIONS

1. Heat the oil in a large nonstick skillet over medium-high heat. Season the steaks with 1/4 tsp salt and the pepper, then add to the skillet. Cook the steaks about 3 minutes on the first side and 2 minutes on the other side for medium-rare meat. Place the steaks on a serving platter.

MORE THAN FOUR?

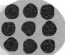

If you want to prepare this steak for eight, double all of the ingredients, but keep the doubled ingredients separate. Use two large sauté pans to prepare the 4-steak batches separately. This might be a good way to have a his vs. hers contest to determine who cooks better steaks.

2. Melt the butter in the same skillet over medium heat. Sauté the green onion, garlic, and rosemary for 30 seconds. Add the wine, broth, and remaining salt and increase the heat to high. Cook for 3 minutes or until the sauce is reduced to about 1/2 cup. Pour the sauce over the steaks and serve immediately.

Exchanges: 4 lean meat; 210 calories, 60 calories from fat, 7 g total fat, 2 g saturated fat, 50 mg cholesterol, 370 mg sodium, 2 g total carbohydrate, 0 g dietary fiber, 0 g sugars, 25 g protein.

⮕ FAST FIX

Befriend your butcher . . . ask her or him to cut your steaks for you. It can save you time and an extra cutting board. But if you don't have a butcher buddy, buy two 8-oz steaks rather than a roast. Simply trim the fat and cut each steak in half.

FOOD FLAIR

Eye of round steak is a very lean cut of beef. It's wonderful when served medium rare. However, it becomes tougher the longer it's cooked using this method. So, if you prefer your beef cooked medium, medium well, or well done, use beef tenderloin instead. It has a little more fat, but it's still considered a lean meat. And it'll still be tender when cooked longer.

TOMATO-GLAZED MEAT LOAF

Serves 4/serving size: 1 slice

Meat loaf has always been a family favorite, though people are often reluctant to admit it. This recipe will become a favorite to make, too—especially if you're the artsy type. "Finger-painting" is required to prepare it. And yes, you can eat the meat loaf "paint"!

- 1 lb lean meat loaf mix, or combine 1/3 lb each ground beef sirloin, veal, and turkey breast (antibiotic free)
- 1 cup minced red onion
- 1 large egg, slightly beaten
- 1/3 cup dry old-fashioned oats
- 1/3 cup organic ketchup (divided use)
- 3 Tbsp spicy honey mustard (divided use)
- 1 tsp finely chopped fresh thyme leaves
- 1/2 tsp garlic salt
- 1/2 tsp freshly ground black pepper, or to taste
- 1/4 tsp ground cinnamon

DIRECTIONS

1. Preheat the oven to 400°F. In a medium bowl, add the meat loaf mix, onion, egg, oats, 2 Tbsp ketchup, 2 Tbsp mustard, thyme, garlic salt, pepper, and cinnamon. Combine well with your hands. Sculpt the mixture into a football-like loaf or other fun shape. Place on a nonstick baking pan.

2. Stir the remaining ketchup and mustard together in a small bowl; this is the "paint." Finger-paint or brush the paint over the top (or top and sides) of the loaf. Bake for 45 minutes or until fully cooked.

3. Let sit 10 minutes before slicing, then cut into 4 slices. Garnish with fresh thyme sprigs, if desired.

Exchanges: 1 carbohydrate, 3 lean meat; 250 calories, 72 calories from fat, 8 g total fat, 2 g saturated fat, 120 mg cholesterol, 550 mg sodium, 17 g total carbohydrate, 2 g dietary fiber, 9 g sugars, 27 g protein.

FRESH FACT

Fresh is usually best. But there are some processed foods that can provide as much or more nutritional benefit than the fresh version. Ketchup is one of those foods. It's a tasty tomato product that, due to its concentration, has a high level of lycopene, a carotenoid antioxidant. A meal plan rich in tomatoes and tomato products containing lycopene has been found to help protect against chronic diseases.

FAST FIX

Don't spend too much time hunting at the supermarket for hot or spicy honey mustard. If you can't easily find it, use regular honey mustard and stir a few drops of hot pepper sauce into it.

FOOD FLAIR

What's in a name? Well, if you don't like the name "meat loaf," try this on for size: "Roasted Beef, Veal, and Turkey Pâté." In fact, that's what this meat loaf is. Oui, it does sound French. But, after all, the basis of many of our recipes and traditional cooking techniques is French—even in this all-American favorite.

JAMAICAN PORK TENDERLOIN ROAST

Serves 4/serving size: 6 slices

One of the most pleasurable ways to eat lean meat is to pair it with fruit. Here, a small amount of tropical fruit juice goes a long way, adding unique flavor, succulence, and a little boost of antioxidants.

- 16 oz lean pork tenderloin, well trimmed (antibiotic free)
- 1/2 cup plus 3 Tbsp apricot, peach, papaya, or mango nectar, not from concentrate (divided use)
- 1/3 cup thinly sliced green onion
- 3 Tbsp naturally brewed reduced-sodium soy sauce
- 1 1/2 tsp canola oil
- 1 Tbsp grated fresh ginger root
- 1/4 tsp ground cinnamon
- 1/4 tsp hot red pepper sauce

DIRECTIONS

1. Place the pork in a large sealable plastic bag. In a medium bowl, whisk together 1/2 cup nectar, green onion, soy sauce, oil, ginger root, cinnamon, and hot pepper sauce. Pour the mixture into the bag, seal tightly, and refrigerate at least 4 hours or overnight, rotating bag occasionally.

2. Preheat the oven to 450°F. Place the marinated pork directly on a nonstick baking pan. Discard the bag and marinade. Roast for 20 minutes or until cooked through, but very slightly pink in the middle. Let stand at least 5 minutes before slicing.

3. Cut the pork into 24 slices. Fan out 6 slices per plate. Drizzle with remaining nectar and garnish with minced or thinly sliced green onion, if desired.

Exchanges: 3 lean meat; 150 calories, 39 calories from fat, 4 g total fat, 2 g saturated fat, 65 mg cholesterol, 160 mg sodium, 3 g total carbohydrate, 0 g dietary fiber, 3 g sugars, 23 g protein.

FAST FIX

Split up cooking techniques. First, pan-sear the roast in a large oven-safe skillet. Then finish roasting in the oven. It'll save a little time and add a little extra flavor from the browning.

FOOD FLAIR

Grill it! Heat the grill over medium heat. Remove the pork from the marinade and discard the marinade. Grill the pork until brown on all sides and very slightly pink in the middle. The grill marks formed on the pork will create a more beautiful presentation— and add that outdoor-cooked goodness.

TUSCAN TURKEY MEATBALLS WITH TORN BASIL

Serves 6/serving size: 3 meatballs

Tuscan cuisine is the original peasant cuisine of Italy. Some notable Tuscan ingredients—parmesan cheese, basil, and wheat—are all used in these lean, yet luscious, meatballs. The torn basil provides a simple, rustic touch.

- 1/2 cup plain whole wheat panko bread crumbs (see Fresh Fact)
- 1/2 cup grated red onion
- 1/2 cup freshly grated Parmigiana-Reggiano cheese
- 1 cup packed fresh basil leaves, half finely chopped, half hand torn (divided use)
- 1 large egg, lightly beaten
- 1 large egg white
- 2 large garlic cloves, minced
- 3/4 tsp crushed red pepper flakes
- 1 lb lean ground turkey breast meat (antibiotic free)
- 3/4 tsp sea salt

DIRECTIONS

1. Preheat the oven to 450°F. Stir the bread crumbs and onion together in a medium bowl and let sit at least 5 minutes.

2. One at a time, stir in each additional ingredient except the torn basil, to assure all gets evenly combined and the turkey doesn't get overmixed. Form the mixture into 18 balls (about 2 Tbsp mixture each). Place on a large nonstick baking pan and bake 18 minutes or until well done. Serve topped with the torn basil.

Exchanges: 1/2 carbohydrate, 2 lean meat; 160 calories, 37 calories from fat, 4 g total fat, 1 g saturated fat, 70 mg cholesterol, 460 mg sodium, 7 g total carbohydrate, 1 g dietary fiber, 1 g sugars, 24 g protein.

FRESH FACT

No worries if you don't have panko bread crumbs. This recipe works well with a scant 1/2 cup of regular whole wheat bread crumbs instead. Wanna make them yourself? Toast whole wheat bread slices in a 250°F oven until the bread is completely dry and crisp. Then grate in a food processor.

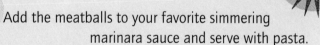

FOOD FLAIR

Add the meatballs to your favorite simmering marinara sauce and serve with pasta.

MORE THAN FOUR?

This recipe can be served as an hors d'oeuvre for 18— one meatball per person. Or it can be easily doubled to serve 12 as an entrée; 36 as an hors d'oeuvre.

SZECHWAN TEMPEH VEGETABLE STIR-FRY

Serves 4/serving size: 1 1/2 cups

Stir-frying is a healthy cooking technique. But often at Chinese restaurants, extra oil can sneak into a stir-fry, adding unnecessary calories and fat. Here you'll know exactly what you're getting. Two teaspoons of flavorful sesame oil goes surprisingly far.

- 3/4 cup natural vegetable broth
- 1/4 cup organic ketchup
- 2 Tbsp naturally brewed reduced-sodium soy sauce
- 2 Tbsp Asian garlic–chili sauce
- 1 1/2 tsp grated fresh ginger root
- 2 tsp toasted sesame oil
- 8 oz tempeh, cut into 24 pieces
- 1 1/2 cups sliced Vidalia, Maui, or other sweet onion
- 3 cups bite-size broccoli florets
- 3 cups sliced red bell pepper

DIRECTIONS

1. In a small saucepan over medium-high heat, add the broth, ketchup, soy sauce, chili sauce, and ginger. Cook for 5 minutes, stirring occasionally.

2. Meanwhile, heat the oil in an extra-large nonstick skillet or wok over medium-high heat. (Reduce the heat if the oil begins to smoke.) Stir-fry the tempeh and onion for 5 minutes or until the tempeh is lightly browned. Add the broccoli and bell peppers and stir-fry for 2 minutes.

3. Add the broth mixture and continue to stir-fry for 1 minute, or until vegetables are tender-crisp. Serve over steamed brown basmati rice or whole wheat couscous.

Exchanges: 1 1/2 carbohydrate, 1 medium-fat meat; 190 calories, 53 calories from fat, 6 g total fat, 1 g saturated fat, 0 mg cholesterol, 480 mg sodium, 20 g total carbohydrate, 8 g dietary fiber, 7 g sugars, 15 g protein.

FRESH FACT

Tempeh is a fermented soybean cake. It looks a little like a weird crispy rice cereal treat. But it's the type of cake that's savory, not sweet. With its dense, chewy texture, it works well in place of meat in this stir-fry. And with its chameleon-like ability to take on taste, the Asian flavors will shine through. Look for it in the refrigerated section of the grocery store.

FAST FIX

Prepare the Szechwan sauce (the first recipe step) up to 3 days in advance. Pour into your own bottle, seal, label, and chill.

FOOD FLAIR

For added flavor, color, and crunch, stir in thinly sliced green onion and finely chopped roasted peanuts just before serving.

BOTTOMLESS BURRITO BOWL

Serves 4/serving size: 1 1/2 cups

Don't worry about overdoing it on carbs with this tasty burrito. It's tortilla-less. And, it's packed with soluble fiber from the beans which may help manage blood glucose.

- 1 (15-oz) can organic black or kidney beans, drained
- 1 medium jalapeño pepper with seeds, thinly sliced crosswise
- 1 Tbsp lime juice (from 1/2 lime)
- 2 cups cooked brown basmati rice, warm or chilled
- 1/4 cup finely chopped fresh cilantro
- 1/2 tsp sea salt, or to taste
- 1/3 cup thinly sliced green onion (slice on diagonal)
- 1 large vine-ripened tomato, seeded and diced (1 cup)
- 1 Hass avocado, peeled and diced (1 cup)
- 1/2 cup natural salsa (mild, medium, or hot)
- 4 small lime wedges (from 1/2 lime)

DIRECTIONS

1. Lightly coat a large nonstick skillet with natural cooking spray and place over medium-high heat. Add the beans and jalapeño and cook, stirring, for 2 minutes. Add the lime juice, rice, cilantro, and salt and stir for 2 minutes or until the rice is hot.

2. Spoon 1 cup of the bean–rice mixture into 4 serving bowls. Top each with green onion, tomato, and avocado. Serve with salsa and lime wedges.

Exchanges: 1 1/2 starch, 2 vegetable, 1 fat; 290 calories, 69 calories from fat, 8 g total fat, 1 g saturated fat, 0 mg cholesterol, 540 mg sodium, 49 g total carbohydrate, 10 g dietary fiber, 6 g sugars, 9 g protein.

FRESH FACT

Better sex is why the Aztecs supposedly loved the avocado—the "forbidden fruit." It's also called the "alligator pear." But most Americans love its luscious texture, taste, and versatility regardless of its name or reputation. The Hass avocado is the most popular of California's seven varieties. And it's popular among nutritionists as well, for its heart-protective monounsaturated fat, fiber, vitamin E, folate, potassium, and other beneficial nutrients.

FAST FIX

Cook the rice a couple of days in advance and refrigerate it. Or cook it up to a couple of months in advance and freeze it.

MORE THAN FOUR?

This bowl is super-easy to serve for 8, 12, 16, or more. To save time, rather than serving individually, place in an extra large salad bowl and have people make their own bowls. If you're making this in advance for a gathering, gently toss diced avocado with fresh lime juice to help prevent browning.

FOOD FLAIR

For added excitement, accessorize your serving with additional toppings, such as diced, grilled chicken breast or flank steak, organic low-fat sour cream, and a sprinkle of Monterey Jack cheese. And, for a unique presentation, serve in bowls made from scooped out iceberg lettuce halves. Shred the scooped out portion of lettuce and use as an ingredient, too.

ROASTED WILD SALMON FILET WITH ORANGE–MISO SAUCE

Serves 4/serving size: 1 filet plus 3 Tbsp sauce

Salmon provides a significant amount of beneficial omega-3 fats. So, don't worry if the total fat content of this entrée is higher than usual. Your heart will thank you. Your taste buds will, too.

- 1 (5.3-oz) container fat-free Greek yogurt or 1/2 cup yogurt cheese (see recipe, page 63)
- 1 1/2 tsp orange zest (grated peel; divided use)
- 3 Tbsp orange juice
- 1 Tbsp mellow white miso
- 2 tsp Dijon mustard
- 1 tsp grated fresh ginger root
- 1/4 tsp toasted sesame oil
- 1/4 tsp sea salt, or to taste
- 16 oz Alaskan Wild King salmon center-cut filet with skin, cut into 4 (4-oz) portions
- 2 tsp naturally brewed reduced-sodium soy sauce
- 2 Tbsp finely chopped pine nuts

DIRECTIONS

1. Preheat the oven to 400°F. In a medium bowl, whisk the yogurt, 3/4 tsp zest, orange juice, miso, mustard, ginger, oil, and salt and set aside.

2. Line a large baking sheet with parchment paper. Place the salmon on the sheet, skin side down. Brush the salmon with soy sauce and pat nuts onto the salmon with your fingers. Roast uncovered for 10 minutes or until done as desired.

3. Spoon the Orange–Miso Sauce onto 4 plates. Place the salmon on top of the sauce and sprinkle with remaining orange zest.

Exchanges: 1/2 carbohydrate, 4 lean meat; 250 calories, 98 calories from fat, 11 g total fat, 1 g saturated fat, 70 mg cholesterol, 480 mg sodium, 6 g total carbohydrate, 2 g dietary fiber, 4 g sugars, 30 g protein.

FRESH FACT

Choose wild salmon instead of farm-raised. It may have less polychlorinated biphenyls (PCBs) and other possible contaminants.

FAST FIX

The Orange-Miso Sauce can be made 1 day in advance. Cover and refrigerate. Bring to room temperature before serving.

FOOD FLAIR

Instead of chopping the pine nuts, leave them whole—2 Tbsp of them. Pan-toast and set aside. Roast the salmon without the pine nuts. Then, on each plate, serve roasted salmon drizzled with Orange-Miso Sauce and sprinkled with toasted pine nuts.

ASIAN SESAME-CRUSTED TUNA STEAK ON ARUGULA

Serves 4/serving size: 1 steak on 1 cup arugula

Normally the word "tuna" conjures up images of a can. But this luscious, yet lean, tuna entrée is so beautifully presented with its black and white sesame seeds, you'll be fine-dining at home—no can included.

- 3 Tbsp rice vinegar
- 1 1/2 Tbsp naturally brewed reduced-sodium soy sauce
- 1 Tbsp honey mustard
- 1/2 tsp toasted sesame oil
- 1 tsp grated fresh ginger root
- 1 small garlic clove, minced
- 4 (4-oz) fresh Wild Yellowfin or Tobago Wild Blackfin tuna steaks (about 1 inch thick)
- 1 (5-oz) package organic baby arugula or 1 bunch fresh arugula, chopped
- 1/4 tsp sea salt, or to taste
- 1/4 cup mixture of black and white sesame seeds

DIRECTIONS

1. In a small bowl, whisk the vinegar, soy sauce, mustard, oil, ginger, and garlic. Using about 2 Tbsp of this vinaigrette, brush the entire surface of the tuna steaks. Toss the remaining vinaigrette with the arugula.

2. Heat a large nonstick skillet over medium-high heat. Sprinkle the tuna with salt. Pour the sesame seeds on a plate and dip each tuna steak into the seeds to coat all sides. Lightly coat steaks with natural cooking spray and cook for 2 minutes per side or until medium-rare. (Reduce the heat to medium if the seeds begin to burn.)

3. Place equal portions (about 1 cup) of argula onto each of 4 plates and top each with a tuna steak.

Exchanges: 1/2 carbohydrate, 3 lean meat; 200 calories, 54 calories from fat, 6 g total fat, 1 g saturated fat, 50 mg cholesterol, 460 mg sodium, 6 g total carbohydrate, 2 g dietary fiber, 2 g sugars, 29 g protein.

FRESH FACT

Ginger, garlic, and mustard add flavor to foods. But they also may provide helpful physiological effects, including playing a beneficial role in diabetes management. So spice it up.

FOOD FLAIR

Slice tuna steaks on the bias (angle) and fan out over the dressed arugula. Thinly slice a scallion on the bias and use as a garnish.

FAST FIX

Unless you're lucky enough to have a friendly neighborhood fishmonger, you might not be able to easily purchase perfect 4-oz tuna steaks. If that's the case, purchase two 8-oz pieces or one 16-oz piece and cut your own individual steaks. And remember this . . . tuna is tastier when cooked a little, not a lot. So it's a time-saving food any way you slice it.

ON THE SIDE

LEMON-ZESTED BROWN RICE PILAF WITH PISTACHIOS

Serves 4/serving size: 3/4 cup

The rich flavor of butter is nearly irreplaceable. Unfortunately, its saturated fat grams can add up quickly. So, choose just enough butter to give you flavor when you need it. This pistachio-studded pilaf balances a just-right amount of butter with full-flavored olive oil— a lower saturated fat choice. You'll still have full flavor enjoyment.

- 1 tsp extra virgin olive oil
- 1 tsp unsalted butter
- 1 large shallot, minced
- 1 cup brown basmati or long-grain brown rice
- 1/4 cup unsalted pistachios, finely chopped (divided use)
- 2 cups natural fat-free chicken or vegetable broth
- 2 Tbsp lemon juice
- 1 tsp lemon zest (grated peel)
- 1/2 tsp sea salt, or to taste

DIRECTIONS

1. Add the oil and butter to a large saucepan over medium heat. Once the butter melts, add the shallot and sauté for 1 minute. Add the rice and 2 Tbsp pistachios. Cook, stirring, for 1 minute.

2. Increase the heat to high. Add the broth and lemon juice and bring to a boil. Reduce the heat to low, cover, and simmer for 50 minutes, or until the liquid is absorbed and the rice is tender.

3. Remove from heat and stir in the lemon zest and salt. Sprinkle with 2 Tbsp pistachios.

Exchanges: 2 1/2 starch, 1 fat; 220 calories, 62 calories from fat, 7 g total fat, 1 g saturated fat, 5 mg cholesterol, 475 mg sodium, 36 g total carbohydrate, 3 g dietary fiber, 2 g sugars, 7 g protein.

FRESH FACT

Zest is the fragrant outermost colored portion of the lemon (or other citrus fruit) skin. For best results, grate it with a Microplane® grater. Just be sure to grate the peel like grated parmesan cheese, with short, sharp strokes, and not peel it like a carrot. And remember that just a small grated amount flavors an entire dish, whether a savory pilaf or a sweet treat.

FOOD FLAIR

Have fun with your food: vary the fruits and nuts in this pilaf. For instance, try orange juice and zest instead of lemon, or almonds instead of pistachios.

VEGGIE FRIED BROWN RICE

Serves 4/serving size: 3/4 cup

Fried rice from your local Chinese carryout—filled with excess sodium and fat—is a diabetes meal plan disaster. But there's no need to forgo this "fried" side. This recipe is naturally healthful and flavorful, since it starts with whole grain rice and is surprisingly full of veggies.

- 1 Tbsp toasted sesame oil
- 1/2 cup thinly sliced green onion
- 1 Tbsp grated fresh ginger root
- 1 cup fresh mung bean sprouts
- 3/4 cup peeled shredded carrot
- 2 cups cooked brown basmati or long-grain brown rice, chilled
- 1/2 cup frozen peas
- 1 1/2 Tbsp naturally brewed reduced-sodium soy sauce, or to taste
- 1 tsp Asian garlic–chili sauce, or to taste
- 1 large egg, lightly beaten

DIRECTIONS

1. Heat the oil in a large nonstick skillet or wok over medium-high heat. Stir-fry the green onion and ginger for 1 minute. Add the sprouts and carrot and stir-fry for 1 minute. Add the chilled rice, frozen peas, soy sauce, and chili sauce. Stir-fry for 2 minutes or until the rice and peas are heated through.

2. Slowly stir the egg into the rice and cook until the egg is scrambled into small pieces and begins to brown. Serve immediately with extra soy sauce on the side. Garnish with additional sliced green onion, if desired. Enjoy with chopsticks.

Exchanges: 2 starch, 1 fat; 200 calories, 52 calories from fat, 6 g total fat, 1 g saturated fat, 55 mg cholesterol, 340 mg sodium, 31 g total carbohydrate, 4 g dietary fiber, 4 g sugars, 7 g protein.

FRESH FACT

A little bit of highly fragrant oil, like toasted sesame, hot chili, white truffle, or extra virgin olive oil, goes a long way, as you'll discover in this delish dish.

FOOD FLAIR

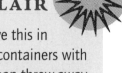

For fun, serve this in takeout containers with chopsticks. Cheap throw-away chopsticks work just as well as expensive ones, too.

MORE THAN FOUR?

You've no doubt heard of refried beans. Well, how about refried rice? Make this recipe 1 day in advance. Re-stir-fry it in a nonstick pan or wok over medium-high heat until it's heated through and begins to lightly crisp. When you double this recipe, re-stir-frying is the best way to serve 8—or more.

HERBED ZUCCHINI—CARROT COUSCOUS STACK

Serves 4/serving size: 1 cup

Think it takes time to create a healthful, flavorful side dish? Think again. Couscous is one of the quickest-cooking grain-based foods because it's already parboiled.

- 1 Tbsp extra virgin olive oil
- 2 large garlic cloves, minced
- 1 1/2 cups natural vegetable broth
- 1 medium zucchini, sliced vertically, then thinly sliced crosswise
- 1/3 cup grated carrot
- 1 cup whole wheat couscous
- 1/4 cup thinly sliced fresh basil leaves
- 2 Tbsp finely chopped fresh oregano
- 1/2 tsp sea salt, or to taste

DIRECTIONS

1. Heat the oil in a medium saucepan over medium heat. Sauté the garlic for 1 1/2 minutes (but don't let it brown). Increase the heat to high and add the broth, zucchini, and carrot. Bring to a boil.

2. Pour in the couscous, giving the mixture a quick stir. Immediately cover with a lid and remove from heat. Let sit for 7 minutes, covered. Then remove the lid and stir in the basil, oregano, and salt.

3. Arrange in 4 stacks by firmly packing the still-hot couscous into a dry measuring cup or circular mold shape. Invert each cup (or carefully remove the circular mold) onto a dinner plate or small individual serving dish. Garnish the top of each stack with fresh basil or an oregano sprig, if desired. Enjoy warm.

Exchanges: 1 1/2 starch, 1 vegetable, 1/2 fat; 160 calories, 39 calories from fat, 4 g total fat, 1 g saturated fat, 0 mg cholesterol, 470 mg sodium, 28 g total carbohydrate, 5 g dietary fiber, 2 g sugars, 5 g protein.

FRESH FACT

In America, couscous is considered a type of pasta. But in many countries it's treated as a grain. It's a wonderful base for highly flavored ingredients and is delicious served warm as a side or cold in a texture-filled, vitamin-packed salad.

FOOD FLAIR

Traditionally, couscous is served topped with stew. So, try this recipe with Simmered Lamb and Vegetable Stew (see recipe, page 174) or another one of your favorites.

FAST FIX

Make this couscous side a day or two in advance. Store it in the refrigerator, then serve as a chilled side salad, not as a stack. If you plan to serve it cool instead of warm, use 1 1/4 cups broth instead of 1 1/2 cups; this will result in slightly fluffier couscous. And, if desired, squirt with lemon juice for added freshness.

FOOD FLAIR

Finely dice a red or yellow bell pepper and add it along with the zucchini and carrots. Also, shred or finely dice zucchini instead of slicing it for a different look in these stacks.

BELL PEPPER QUINOA PILAF WITH FRESH BASIL

Serves 4/serving size: rounded 1/2 cup

Quinoa, pronounced KEEN-wah, is a whole grain. It's also considered a "supergrain," as it's higher in protein than all other grains. It's slightly lower in carbohydrates than most grains, too. That makes quinoa uniquely fit for a diabetes meal plan—or any meal plan.

- 1 cup quinoa
- 2 cups spring water
- 1 cup finely diced red bell pepper
- 1 Tbsp fresh lemon juice
- 3/4 tsp sea salt, or to taste
- 1 1/2 tsp extra virgin olive oil
- 1/3 cup thinly sliced or finely chopped fresh basil leaves
- 2 Tbsp pine nuts, pan-toasted

DIRECTIONS

1. Bring the quinoa, water, bell pepper, lemon juice, and salt to a boil in a medium saucepan over high heat. Reduce the heat to medium, cover, and simmer for 12 minutes or until the water is absorbed and the quinoa is tender. Remove from the heat.

2. Stir in the olive oil and about 3/4 of the basil. Transfer to a serving bowl and top with the remaining basil and pine nuts.

Exchanges: 2 starch, 1 vegetable, 1 fat; 210 calories, 65 calories from fat, 7 g total fat, 1 g saturated fat, 0 mg cholesterol, 440 mg sodium, 33 g total carbohydrate, 3 g dietary fiber, 1 g sugars, 7 g protein.

FOOD FLAIR

For more highly flavored quinoa,
use natural vegetable broth for simmering
instead of water. Just use less salt to account for
the sodium in the broth. And for more eye
appeal, use half red and half yellow bell pepper.

FRESH FACT

Many whole grains can take 45 minutes or longer to prepare.
Quinoa is an exception—it cooks in less than 15 minutes.

FAST FIX

Prepare this light and fluffy pilaf up to
2 days in advance. Cover and refrigerate,
then serve chilled with lemon wedges.

STEWED ROSEMARY BEAN BED

Serves 4/serving size: 1/2 cup

These beans are so creamy they'll practically melt in your mouth. Serve these as a bed for roasted chicken, duck, or any lean roasted meat. Round out the meal with a rich-tasting, texture-filled veggie, like Brussels sprouts or broccoli.

- 2 tsp extra virgin olive oil
- 2 medium leeks, white and pale green parts only, halved vertically and thinly sliced horizontally
- 1 (15-oz) can organic Great Northern or other white beans, drained
- 3/4 cup natural vegetable broth
- 1/2 tsp minced fresh rosemary

DIRECTIONS

1. Heat the oil in a large saucepan over medium heat. Add the leeks and cook, stirring frequently, for 5 minutes or until the leeks are softened (but don't let them brown).

2. Add the beans, broth, and rosemary and bring to a full boil over high heat. Reduce the heat to medium and simmer for 5 minutes, or until the liquid is nearly evaporated.

Exchanges: 1 starch, 1/2 fat; 90 calories, 23 calories from fat, 3 g total fat, 0 g saturated fat, 0 mg cholesterol, 160 mg sodium, 15 g total carbohydrate, 4 g dietary fiber, 3 g sugars, 4 g protein.

FRESH FACT

After slicing the leeks, add them to a bowl of water, swish around, rinse, and drain well before using. Otherwise, they'll be gritty and ruin this lovely side.

FOOD FLAIR

Garnish each serving with a fresh rosemary sprig to add a special touch. Vary the taste, texture, and look by experimenting with different beans and herbs. Kick up the flavor by adding 1/8 tsp crushed red pepper flakes with the broth.

SOUTHWESTERN CILANTRO–LIME PINTOS

Serves 4/serving size: scant 1/2 cup

Trying to find a flavorful (and fast!) way to add fiber to your meal plan? Look no further. One word describes these beans: yum!

- 2 tsp peanut or canola oil
- 1 large garlic clove, minced
- 1 small jalapeño pepper with some seeds, minced
- 1 (15-oz) can organic pinto beans, drained
- 1/4 cup natural vegetable broth
- 1/4 cup chopped fresh cilantro
- 1 Tbsp lime juice

DIRECTIONS

1. Heat the oil in a medium saucepan over medium-high heat. Add the garlic and jalapeño and cook, stirring, for 30 seconds. Add the beans and broth and cook, stirring occasionally, for 3 minutes or until the liquid is nearly evaporated.

2. Remove from the heat and stir in the cilantro and lime juice. Serve hot as a side or cool as a salad.

Exchanges: 1 starch; 80 calories, 20 calories from fat, 2 g total fat, 0 g saturated fat, 0 mg cholesterol, 105 mg sodium, 11 g total carbohydrate, 4 g dietary fiber, 1 g sugars, 3 g protein.

FOOD FLAIR

If you're serving these beans hot, lightly top them with shredded Monterey Jack cheese immediately after stirring in the cilantro and lime juice. For a more substantial side—or perhaps an entrée—stir the Southwestern Cilantro-Lime Pintos into steamed brown rice.

HARICOT VERTS AMANDINE

Serves 4/serving size: scant 1 cup

"Haricot verts" is French for green string beans. So not only are these savory beans skinny, the entire side dish is skinny—at just 60 calories a serving. Best of all, these beans are rich in fiber. So they'll fill you up while helping to keep your weight down and blood glucose steady.

- 1 lb fresh green beans, preferably haricot verts, trimmed
- 1 tsp unsalted butter
- 1/4 cup water
- 2 tsp fresh lemon juice
- 1/4 tsp sea salt, or to taste
- 1/8 tsp freshly ground black pepper, or to taste
- 1 Tbsp sliced almonds, pan-toasted

DIRECTIONS

1. Place the beans, butter, and water in an extra-large skillet over medium-high heat. Cook, uncovered, while tossing with tongs, for 5 minutes or until the water is evaporated and the beans are tender-crisp and bright green. (If the beans begin to brown, reduce the heat.)

2. Add the lemon juice and toss for 30 seconds, then remove from heat. Sprinkle with salt, pepper, and almonds.

Exchanges: 2 vegetable, 1/2 fat; 60 calories, 18 calories from fat, 2 g total fat, 1 g saturated fat, 5 mg cholesterol, 150 mg sodium, 9 g total carbohydrate, 4 g dietary fiber, 2 g sugars, 2 g protein.

FRESH FACT

Almonds are the richest nut source of calcium and they're loaded with heart-protective vitamin E. The average American diet doesn't contain enough of either nutrient. A little sprinkle of almonds here and there—like in this easy, yet impressive, side dish—can be the delicious answer to this dietary dilemma.

MINTY PETITE PEAS

Serves 4/serving size: scant 1/2 cup

Peas have suffered from an image problem in the past. But this tasty, simple recipe is sure to put them back in your good graces. The hint of fresh mint in these sweet peas makes them a palate-pleasing accompaniment to lamb, salmon, or shrimp.

- 1 (10-oz) package frozen petite or baby peas
- 2 Tbsp water
- 2 tsp finely chopped fresh mint
- 2 tsp unsalted butter
- 1/2 tsp sea salt, or to taste

DIRECTIONS

Place all ingredients in a medium saucepan and cook over medium heat, stirring constantly, for 5 minutes or until hot. Garnish each serving with a fresh mint sprig, if desired.

Exchanges: 1/2 starch, 1/2 fat; 70 calories, 18 calories from fat, 2 g total fat, 1 g saturated fat, 5 mg cholesterol, 340 mg sodium, 10 g total carbohydrate, 4 g dietary fiber, 3 g sugars, 4 g protein.

FRESH FACT

At a farmers' market, you might have a choice between fresh peppermint and spearmint. Pick the peppermint—it's more pungent.

FOOD FLAIR

Mix leftovers (if you ever have any!) into cooked whole wheat couscous or brown rice for a palate-pleasing combination—and a satiating side.

FOOD FLAIR

For a change of taste, try fresh tarragon instead of mint. Then pair the peas with chicken.

ROASTED GARLIC MASHED BABY CREAMER POTATOES

Serves 8/serving size: 1/2 cup

All you really need to say is "wow" to this rustic potato recipe. It's bursting with flavor from the roasted garlic and deceivingly rich. Do use the truffle oil when possible, too. It adds a glorious finish.

- 8 large garlic cloves, peeled
- 1 1/2 tsp extra virgin olive oil
- 2 lb red, purple, or Yukon gold baby creamer potatoes with peel
- 1/2 cup fat-free milk, warm
- 1 tsp unsalted butter
- 1 tsp sea salt, or to taste
- 1/4 tsp freshly ground black pepper, or to taste
- 1 Tbsp white truffle oil or extra virgin olive oil

1. Preheat the oven to 425°F. Place the garlic on a piece of heavy-duty foil and drizzle with oil. Wrap up and roast 20 minutes or until softened. Remove from the oven and let sit, wrapped, for at least 2 minutes before opening.

2. Meanwhile, add potatoes to a large saucepan or stockpot and cover with cold water. Bring to a boil and cook for 20 minutes or until very tender, making sure the potatoes are always submerged in water. Turn off the heat and drain well in a colander. Return the potatoes to the pot.

FRESH FACT

Potatoes can raise your blood glucose level quickly, so keep an eye on your serving size. Enjoy them with a protein-rich entrée for balance.

3. Add roasted garlic with roasting oil (if any remains), milk, butter, salt, and pepper. Mash with a potato masher until smooth, adding additional milk if necessary. Transfer to a serving bowl and drizzle with truffle or olive oil.

Exchanges: 1 1/2 starch, 1/2 fat; 120 calories, 29 calories from fat, 3 g total fat, 1 g saturated fat, 0 mg cholesterol, 300 mg sodium, 20 g total carbohydrate, 2 g dietary fiber, 2 g sugars, 3 g protein.

FAST FIX

If some baby potatoes aren't so baby-sized, it's best to cut them into similar-size pieces—or halve the largest ones for more even cooking. Smaller pieces cook faster, too.

Even if you want potatoes for one, two, or four, go ahead and make this entire batch, then refrigerate or freeze it. Leftovers still taste great reheated in the microwave.

FOOD FLAIR

White truffle oil is typically available in Italian markets, specialty food stores, and some fine quality supermarkets. Some oils might only have truffle flavor or aroma added. For the fullest flavor, go for the real thing—not these cheaper versions. White truffle oil is costly, but a little goes a long way.

SAUTÉED BABY SPINACH WITH CURRANTS AND PINE NUTS

Serves 4/serving size: 1/2 cup

Spinach is one of the most popular vegetables in America. You'll especially enjoy this slightly fruity, slightly nutty version. And at only 80 calories a serving, you can enjoy it often.

- 1 tsp extra virgin olive oil
- 1 large garlic clove, thinly sliced
- 1 lb fresh organic baby spinach
- 1 1/2 Tbsp lemon juice (from 1/2 lemon)

- 1 Tbsp currants
- 1/2 tsp sea salt, or to taste
- 1/8 tsp freshly ground pepper, or to taste

- 1 Tbsp pine nuts, pan-toasted
- 4 lemon wedges (from 1/2 lemon)

DIRECTIONS

1. Heat the oil in an extra-large nonstick skillet over medium heat. Add the garlic and cook, stirring, for 2 minutes or until the garlic just begins to lightly brown. Place the garlic on a small plate.

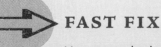

FAST FIX

Use prewashed, prepackaged baby spinach to save valuable time in the kitchen.

2. Add the spinach to the skillet by handfuls. As you add each handful, move the slightly wilted spinach on top of the added leaves. Cook and toss, using tongs with a silicone or nylon head, for 4 minutes or until all the spinach is just wilted.

3. Add the lemon juice and currants and cook, stirring, for 30 seconds. Remove from heat and sprinkle with salt and pepper. Using the tongs, transfer the spinach to a serving bowl or platter. Top with garlic slices and pine nuts and serve with lemon wedges.

Exchanges: 1 carbohydrate; 80 calories, 24 calories from fat, 3 g total fat, 0 g saturated fat, 0 mg cholesterol, 470 mg sodium, 15 g total carbohydrate, 6 g dietary fiber, 2 g sugars, 3 g protein.

FRESH FACT

Spinach is a nutrient-dense food, providing a big bang of nutrients in a small number of calories. One of the key nutrients in spinach is lutein, an antioxidant that may reduce the risk of age-related macular degeneration.

SPRING ASPARAGUS STIR-FRY

Serves 4/serving size: rounded 1 cup

Stir-fries are ideal for sides, not just entrées. Try pairing this amazing asparagus stir-fry with an orange- and ginger-accented roasted salmon or chicken entrée and steamed brown basmati rice. Oh, so good—and good for you.

- 2 Tbsp naturally brewed reduced-sodium soy sauce
- 1 Tbsp acacia or other mild floral honey
- 2 tsp toasted sesame oil

- 2 large garlic cloves, minced
- 1 tsp grated fresh ginger root
- 2 lb asparagus, ends trimmed, cut on diagonal into 2-inch-long pieces

- 1/4 tsp sea salt, or to taste
- 1 tsp sesame seeds, roasted or toasted

DIRECTIONS

1. In a small bowl, stir the soy sauce and honey together and set aside.

FAST FIX

The skinnier, the speedier when it comes to asparagus. So choose the pencil-like asparagus when you can find it. Without thick stems, little trimming is required. And the pieces can be stir-fried all at once—about 2 minutes total.

2. Heat the oil in a large skillet or wok over medium-high heat. (Reduce the heat if the oil begins to smoke.) Add the garlic and ginger and cook, stirring, for 30 seconds.

3. Add the thick-stemmed asparagus pieces and stir-fry for 1 minute. Add the thin-stemmed asparagus pieces and stir-fry for 1 minute. Add the asparagus tips and stir-fry for 2 minutes or until tender-crisp.

4. Add the soy sauce–honey mixture and cook, stirring, for 1 minute or until the asparagus is well coated. Sprinkle with salt. Transfer the asparagus with any remaining sauce to a serving bowl and sprinkle with sesame seeds.

Exchanges: 2 vegetable, 1/2 fat; 80 calories, 26 calories from fat, 3 g total fat, 0 g saturated fat, 0 mg cholesterol, 470 mg sodium, 12 g total carbohydrate, 3 g dietary fiber, 6 g sugars, 5 g protein.

FRESH FACT

You may consider Chinese food off limits if you're watching dietary sodium. So balance higher sodium choices with full-flavored, lower sodium choices. Your best bet is to stick to a Chinese side instead of an entrée, like this appetizing asparagus.

FOOD FLAIR

Asparagus is at its nutritious best in springtime when it's at its peak. But don't just stick with the usual green variety. When you can find it, try white or purple asparagus. The white type is especially tender.

THYMELY CORN ON THE COB

Serves 4/serving size: 1 ear corn plus 1 1/2 tsp butter mixture

Thyme is popular in French cuisine. And corn can be considered an icon of American cuisine. Marry them together and you get a memorable food experience.

- 1/4 cup natural vegetable broth
- 1/4 medium Vidalia, Maui, or other sweet onion, peeled

- 2 tsp unsalted butter
- 1 tsp finely chopped fresh thyme leaves

- 4 (7-inch) ears fresh corn, shucked
- 1/4 tsp sea salt, or to taste

DIRECTIONS

1. Puree the broth and onion in a blender for 1 minute or until the onion is fully pureed.

2. Bring the puree to a boil in a small nonstick skillet over medium-high heat. Cook, stirring, for 3 1/2 minutes or until the mixture is the consistency of applesauce and begins to lightly brown.

3. Stir in the butter and thyme and cook, stirring, for 30 seconds. Pour into a ramekin or very small serving bowl and refrigerate.

4. Add the corn to a large pot of boiling water over high heat. Boil the corn for 5 minutes or until tender. Using tongs, remove to a platter. Serve with the thyme butter and salt.

Exchanges: 1 starch, 1/2 fat; 100 calories, 27 calories from fat, 3 g total fat, 1 g saturated fat, 5 mg cholesterol, 190 mg sodium, 18 g total carbohydrate, 3 g dietary fiber, 4 g sugars, 3 g protein.

FOOD FLAIR

Having a cookout? Grill the corn instead of boiling it. Prepare the grill (use medium-high heat). Grill the corn away from direct heat, rotating frequently, for 8 minutes, or until it's slightly blackened in spots.

FAST FIX

You can prepare the thyme butter up to 2 days in advance. Keep it covered and refrigerated. It's best to bring it to room temperature before using.

MORE THAN FOUR?

Summer is the season for picking corn—and for having parties. Whether you cook out or in, this recipe is an easy winner for 4, 8, 12, or more. For a pretty and playful presentation, tear the outer layer of a few corn husks into strips. Then tie a strip around each cooked ear of corn.

SAGE SWEET POTATO FRITES

Serves 4/serving size: 9 frites

Sweet potatoes are rich in beta-carotene, an antioxidant. Their vivid orange color is a clue to that richness. Try these visually appealing fries as a healthier alternative to French fries. ("Frites" is just the French way of referring to them.) They have a tender texture and unique flavor that's as richly sweet as it is savory.

- 1 Tbsp apple cider vinegar
- 2 tsp unsalted butter, melted
- 1 tsp extra virgin olive oil
- 1 tsp ground sage

- 1 1/2 lb sweet potatoes, peeled and cut into 1/2-inch-wide slices, then 1/2-inch-wide sticks

- 3/4 tsp sea salt, or to taste
- 2 Tbsp finely sliced fresh sage leaves

DIRECTIONS

1. Preheat the oven to 450°F. In small bowl, whisk the vinegar, butter, oil, and sage. Pour into a large sealable plastic bag, add the sweet potato sticks, and toss to coat.

2. Line a large baking sheet with parchment paper and spread the sweet potatoes in a single layer on the paper. Sprinkle with salt and bake for 30 minutes or until the sweet potatoes are cooked through and lightly browned.

3. Transfer the sweet potatoes to a platter and sprinkle with fresh sage.

Exchanges: 1 1/2 starch; 120 calories, 29 calories from fat, 3 g total fat, 1 g saturated fat, 5 mg cholesterol, 470 mg sodium, 22 g total carbohydrate, 3 g dietary fiber, 7 g sugars, 2 g protein.

FRESH FACT

There are two types of sweet potatoes—a pale-skinned and a darker-skinned variety. Many people often call the darker-skinned variety a yam. But the yam is from a completely different plant family. The darker-skinned sweet potato is used most often in this country— the one with the beautiful orange flesh that's moist and sweet. As long as you buy these for this recipe, don't worry if they're labeled "yams" or "sweet potatoes." Just enjoy them!

FOOD FLAIR

Crisp these frites before serving by briefly placing them under the broiler. The browning, or caramelizing, actually makes this root veggie taste sweeter. Then, for an eye-appealing presentation, serve each portion in a stack of crisscrossing layers.

FAST FIX

No parchment paper? No problem. Your sweet potatoes will still survive their oven stay without getting stuck on the pan if you use Silpat® instead. Silpat® is a reusable, nonstick, fiberglass–silicone mat that fits right on your baking pan. It works great for cookies, too. The best part: you can use it hundreds, even thousands of times!

ROSEMARY ROASTED ROOT VEGETABLES

Serves 6/serving size: 2/3 cup

Roasting veggies is a wonderful way to enjoy all of their bountiful benefits in fall and winter. The best part: the scent of rosemary will waft through your home during roasting, which will make these veggies even more enticing.

- 2 large parsnips, peeled and sliced crosswise into 3/4-inch-thick coins
- 1 large turnip, peeled and sliced crosswise into 1-inch-thick pieces, then into wedges
- 1 medium sweet potato, peeled and sliced crosswise into 1-inch-thick pieces, then into half rounds
- 1 1/2 Tbsp extra virgin olive oil (divided use)
- 2 tsp finely chopped fresh rosemary
- 3/4 tsp sea salt, or to taste
- 1 large leek, white and pale green parts only, cut vertically and then into 1-inch-thick half rounds
- 4 large garlic cloves, minced

DIRECTIONS

1. Preheat the oven to 400°F. Add the parsnips, turnip, sweet potato, 1 Tbsp oil, rosemary, and salt to a large bowl or sealable plastic bag and toss to coat.

2. Transfer the vegetables to a large nonstick baking sheet or pan and roast for 20 minutes. Stir in the leeks and roast for 20 minutes more.

3. In a small bowl, combine the garlic with remaining oil. Stir the garlic mixture into the roasted vegetables. Roast for 20 minutes more or until vegetables are tender and lightly browned.

Exchanges: 1 1/2 starch, 1/2 fat; 140 calories, 35 calories from fat, 4 g total fat, 1 g saturated fat, 0 mg cholesterol, 320 mg sodium, 24 g total carbohydrate, 5 g dietary fiber, 8 g sugars, 2 g protein.

FRESH FACT

Choosing a variety of vegetables is one way to assure you're getting a variety of beneficial nutrients—and all at once in this side.

FAST FIX

Roast these veggies in advance. Then place them in a 450°F oven to reheat for 10 minutes, or until fully heated through. This way you'll be able to perfectly time them to serve along with your entrée.

FOOD FLAIR

Try varying this recipe each time you make it. Swap out one of the vegetables for carrots, celery root (celeriac), or beets. It's an easy and enticing way to experience new veggies, too.

REFRESHERS

BLUEBERRY SILKEN SMOOTHIE

Serves 2/serving size: 1 cup

This fruit smoothie contains three of the healthiest ingredients ever—blueberries, cranberries, and soy. And it still tastes great!

- 1 1/2 cups fresh blueberries, frozen (or use store-bought frozen berries)
- 2/3 cup organic cranberry juice, chilled
- 3 oz soft silken tofu, drained and chilled (about 1/3 cup)
- 1/8 tsp pure vanilla extract (optional)

DIRECTIONS

Puree all ingredients in a blender on low speed for 30 seconds, then high speed for 30 seconds or until smooth. Serve in chilled glasses.

Exchanges: 1 1/2 carbohydrate; 120 calories, 13 calories from fat, 2 g total fat, 0 g saturated fat, 0 mg cholesterol, 10 mg sodium, 25 g total carbohydrate, 3 g dietary fiber, 20 g sugars, 3 g protein.

FRESH FACT

In general, the richer the color, the more plentiful the nutrients. This smoothie's vivid purple color with deep blue flecks is a sure sign of good nutrition.

FOOD FLAIR

Experiment with various berries and real fruit juices—the combinations are nearly endless.

STRAWBERRY–BANANA SMOOTHIE

Serves 2/serving size: 1 cup

Sip this carb-heavy smoothie along with a carb-light meal, such as a salad topped with grilled chicken. You can enjoy this delicious, refreshing, 100% fruit recipe in any season.

- 1 cup whole fresh strawberries, frozen (or use store-bought whole frozen strawberries)
- 1 medium banana, peeled, frozen, and cut into chunks
- 1 cup organic unsweetened apple juice, chilled

DIRECTIONS

1. Puree the strawberries, banana, and juice in a blender on low speed for 30 seconds, then high speed for 30 seconds or until smooth.

2. Serve in chilled glasses. Garnish with fresh strawberries wedged on glass rims, if desired.

Exchanges: 2 fruit; 130 calories, 5 calories from fat, 1 g total fat, 0 g saturated fat, 0 mg cholesterol, 0 mg sodium, 32 g total carbohydrate, 3 g dietary fiber, 23 g sugars, 1 g protein.

FAST FIX

Peel, cut, and freeze banana slices in small, sealable freezer bags—1 banana per bag. You can freeze them up to several weeks. And you can freeze your own strawberries— 1 cup fresh strawberries per freezer bag.

TRIPLE CHOCOLATE SOY SMOOTHIE

Serves 2/serving size: 3/4 cup

The word "smoothie" has become the modern word for "shake." Though smoothies are usually made with fruit, you won't find any in this chocolaty concoction. It's filled with natural silkiness—and extra protein—from soy. So, plan ahead when you want to satisfy your sweet tooth with this carb-rich dessert. Then sip for joy.

- 3/4 cup low-fat chocolate or vanilla-fudge soy frozen dessert, solidly frozen
- 3/4 cup chocolate soy milk, chilled
- 2 tsp unsweetened natural cocoa powder

DIRECTIONS

Puree all ingredients in a blender on low speed for 15 seconds, then high speed for 15 seconds or until smooth. Serve in chilled glasses.

Exchanges: 2 carbohydrate, 1/2 fat; 170 calories, 26 calories from fat, 3 g total fat, 1 g saturated fat, 0 mg cholesterol, 130 mg sodium, 33 g total carbohydrate, 1 g dietary fiber, 22 g sugars, 4 g protein.

FOOD FLAIR

For a thicker smoothie, simply add less soy milk. For a sexy taste twist, blend in 1/8 tsp pure peppermint or almond extract.

COCOA–MINT FROTHY FOR TWO

Serves 2/serving size: 1 cup

This is sort of like a kissably minty chocolate milkshake. But, at only 90 calories a glass, this delectable drink can be consumed regularly, not rarely.

- 8 ice cubes (vary quantity depending on desired consistency)
- 2 Tbsp unsweetened natural cocoa powder
- 1 Tbsp acacia or orange blossom honey
- 2/3 cup low-fat milk
- 1/2 tsp pure vanilla extract
- 1/8 tsp pure peppermint extract

DIRECTIONS

Puree all ingredients in a blender on low speed for 30 seconds, then high speed for 30 seconds or until smooth and frothy. Serve in chilled glasses.

Exchanges: 1 carbohydrate; 90 calories, 12 calories from fat, 1 g total fat, 0 g saturated fat, 5 mg cholesterol, 45 mg sodium, 16 g total carbohydrate, 1 g dietary fiber, 12 g sugars, 4 g protein.

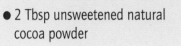

FRESH FACT

Stock up on cocoa powder when it's on sale. When sealed in an airtight container, it can be stored for up to 2 years in a cool, dark place.

FOOD FLAIR

Are you a chocolate purist? Skip the peppermint extract to make a Cocoa Frothy for Two instead.

MANGO LASSI

Serves 2/serving size: 1 cup

This can be considered India's version of the milkshake. It also can be considered one of the thickest, creamiest, most delicious ways to get dairy and fruit all at once.

- 4 large ice cubes (vary quantity depending on desired consistency)
- 1 cup plain low-fat yogurt
- 1 medium mango, peeled and cubed
- 2 tsp turbinado sugar (optional)

DIRECTIONS

Puree all ingredients in a blender on low speed for 30 seconds, then high speed for 30 seconds or until smooth. Serve in tall glasses.

Exchanges: 2 carbohydrate; 150 calories, 19 calories from fat, 2 g total fat, 1 g saturated fat, 5 mg cholesterol, 80 mg sodium, 27 g total carbohydrate, 2 g dietary fiber, 25 g sugars, 7 g protein.

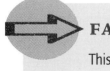

FAST FIX

This drink will keep, covered, up to 3 days in the refrigerator. Whip again before serving.

FOOD FLAIR

If you prefer more sweetness, use the 2 tsp sugar; it adds just enough sweetness to help balance the lassi's yogurt tang. However, you can do it both ways—with and without. Blend the recipe without sugar and pour out 1 cup for yourself. Then add 1 tsp sugar to the rest and blend for a buddy. Or, if you prefer a thinner lassi, add 1 or more tablespoons cold water while blending, until you reach the desired consistency.

AFTER-SCHOOL SIPPER

Serves 2/serving size: 1 1/4 cups

This sensational sipper is a balanced beverage with three food groups in one glass. It can serve as a filling and refreshing after-school snack for kids—or an after-work treat for adults, too.

- 4 large ice cubes (vary quantity depending on desired consistency)
- 2 medium bananas, sliced
- 1 Tbsp natural creamy peanut butter
- 1 cup low-fat milk or vanilla soy milk, chilled

DIRECTIONS

Puree all ingredients in a blender on low speed for 30 seconds, then high speed for 30 seconds or until smooth. Serve in chilled glasses.

Exchanges: 2 1/2 fruit, 1/2 fat-free milk, 1 fat; 230 calories, 52 calories from fat, 6 g total fat, 1 g saturated fat, 5 mg cholesterol, 85 mg sodium, 41 g total carbohydrate, 4 g dietary fiber, 26 g sugars, 6 g protein.

FRESH FACT

Banana slices can act like ice! Just freeze the banana slices in advance, then skip the added ice.

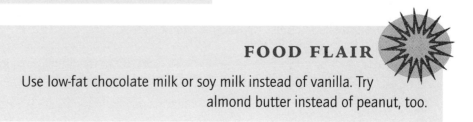

FOOD FLAIR

Use low-fat chocolate milk or soy milk instead of vanilla. Try almond butter instead of peanut, too.

SPARKLING STRAWBERRY–MINT INFUSED WATER

Serves 4/serving size: 1 cup

Quench your thirst with fizzy, flavored H_2O, not just plain ol' H_2O. At just 15 calories, it's not sweet, but it is exceptionally tasty.

- 4 large fresh strawberries, stemmed
- 4 large or 8 small fresh mint leaves
- 2 tsp fresh lemon juice
- 2 tsp turbinado sugar
- 3 1/2 cups sparkling water (divided use)

DIRECTIONS

1. Puree the strawberries, mint, lemon juice, sugar, and 1/2 cup sparkling water in a blender on low speed for 30 seconds or until smooth.

2. Pour the puree into a serving pitcher. Very slowly pour in the remaining sparkling water. Serve chilled over ice.

Exchanges: free; 15 calories, 0 calories from fat, 0 g total fat, 0 g saturated fat, 0 mg cholesterol, 0 mg sodium, 4 g total carbohydrate, 1 g dietary fiber, 3 g sugars, 0 g protein.

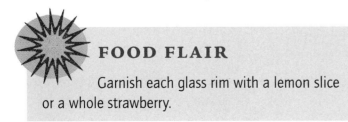

FOOD FLAIR

Garnish each glass rim with a lemon slice or a whole strawberry.

HONEY HOT COCOA AU LAIT

Serves 2/serving size: 3/4 cup

This is hot chocolate for dark chocolate lovers—with just enough sweetness to satisfy. Sip it along with breakfast as a wonderfully warm start to a chilly morning.

- 2 Tbsp unsweetened natural cocoa powder
- 1/4 cup spring water
- 1 1/2 cups low-fat milk
- 1 Tbsp acacia or orange blossom honey
- 1/4 tsp pure vanilla extract

DIRECTIONS

1. Whisk the cocoa and spring water together in a small saucepan over medium heat until the mixture boils. Boil, whisking, for 30 seconds.

2. Pour in the milk and whisk for 3 to 4 minutes or until hot—but don't let the milk boil. Remove from heat, stir in the honey and vanilla, and serve immediately.

Exchanges: 1/2 fat-free milk, 1 carbohydrate, 1/2 fat; 140 calories, 21 calories from fat, 2 g total fat, 1 g saturated fat, 10 mg cholesterol, 100 mg sodium, 21 g total carbohydrate, 1 g dietary fiber, 17 g sugars, 8 g protein.

FOOD FLAIR

Add 1/8 tsp pure almond or peppermint extract. The peppermint actually adds a hint of sweetness without extra sugar. The almond makes it downright nutty!

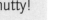

HOMEMADE CHOCOLATE MILK

Serves 4/serving size: 1 cup

Commercial chocolate milk can contain high fructose corn syrup, modified food starch, and artificial flavors—at more than 200 calories a cup. Now you can have your chocolate milk and feel good about it, too.

- 1/4 cup unsweetened natural cocoa powder
- 3 Tbsp turbinado sugar
- 1/8 tsp sea salt
- 1/3 cup spring water
- 3 1/2 cups low-fat milk
- 3/4 tsp pure vanilla extract
- 1/8 tsp pure almond extract (optional)

DIRECTIONS

1. Whisk the cocoa, sugar, salt, and water together in a medium saucepan over medium heat until the mixture boils. Boil, whisking, for 30 seconds.

2. Pour in the milk and whisk for 5 minutes or until hot—but don't let the milk boil.

3. Remove from heat, add vanilla and almond extract (if using), and pour into a heatproof pitcher. Chill. Stir or lightly shake before serving.

Exchanges: 1 fat-free milk, 1/2 carbohydrate, 1/2 fat; 150 calories, 24 calories from fat, 3 g total fat, 1 g saturated fat, 15 mg cholesterol, 190 mg sodium, 23 g total carbohydrate, 1 g dietary fiber, 20 g sugars, 9 g protein.

FRESH FACT

Most of us weaned ourselves off whole milk long ago, down to reduced fat (2%), then low fat (1%) or fat free. Gradually reducing sugar in recipes can be the next step. While 1/4 cup turbinado sugar makes this recipe perfectly sweet for some, 3 Tbsp is also plenty. Over time, you can enjoy this concoction with 2 Tbsp sugar or less. Keep reducing the amount of sugar in your meal plan, just as you did with fat!

PASSION FRUIT MIMOSA WITH RASPBERRIES

Serves 4/serving size: 1 mimosa

It's okay to be passionate about this sparkling passion fruit mimosa made with chilled bubbly … in moderation, of course. Cheers!

- 1/2 cup fresh or frozen raspberries
- 1 1/3 cups sparkling white wine or champagne, chilled
- 3/4 cup passion fruit nectar, chilled

DIRECTIONS

Divide the raspberries among 4 champagne glasses, add the wine or champagne, and top with juice.

Exchanges: 1/2 fruit plus 60 calories from alcohol; 100 calories, 0 calories from fat, 0 g total fat, 0 g saturated fat, 0 mg cholesterol, 0 mg sodium, 10 g total carbohydrate, 1 g dietary fiber, 7 g sugars, 0 g protein.

FOOD FLAIR

Make your mimosa with a variety of nectars, such as mango or apricot.

FRESH FACT

Light to moderate alcohol intake is associated with reduced risk of death due to coronary heart disease for people with type 2 diabetes—great news for some! Moderation is considered one drink a day for women and two for men. And if you do choose to drink, enjoy alcohol with food to minimize unexpected effects on blood glucose levels.

ICED GINGER–PEACH TEA

Serves 4/serving size: 1 cup

Though there are only 15 calories in this refreshing tea, they may not actually count like 15 calories in other beverages. Why? Caffeine in tea may slightly boost the burning of calories, which may help lower body weight. But watch your total daily caffeine intake, which can creep up on you.

- 1 large peach, peeled and sliced
- 4 cups spring water (divided use)
- 1 small piece peeled ginger root (about 1 Tbsp)
- 4 Irish or English Breakfast or other black tea bags

DIRECTIONS

1. Puree the peach slices and 1/2 cup water in a blender until smooth.

2. Bring the puree, remaining water, and ginger root just to a boil in a large saucepan or teapot. Remove from heat and add the tea bags. Let steep for 7 minutes.

3. Remove the tea bags and refrigerate the tea until well chilled. Remove the ginger root and stir before serving over ice.

Exchanges: free; 15 calories, 0 calories from fat, 0 g total fat, 0 g saturated fat, 0 mg cholesterol, 0 mg sodium, 4 g total carbohydrate, 1 g dietary fiber, 3 g sugars, 0 g protein.

FAST FIX

When peaches aren't in season or you
don't want to mess with peeling them, use
3/4 cup frozen sliced peaches instead.

FRESH FACT

Go green! Recent Japanese research found that people who
drink lots of green tea daily may significantly lower their risk
of diabetes. So enjoy this fruity beverage with green tea
instead of black—or do two bags of each.

FOOD FLAIR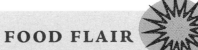

Let people sweeten their own servings
to their individual preferences.

ICED BLUEBERRY EARL GREY TEA

Serves 4/serving size: 1 cup

Running out of healthful, low-calorie beverage options? Add fruit to tea—it's a great way to satisfy your thirst in a naturally interesting alternative.

- 1/2 cup fresh or frozen thawed blueberries
- 4 cups spring water (divided use)
- 4 Earl Grey tea bags

DIRECTIONS

1. Puree the blueberries and 1/2 cup water in a blender until smooth.

2. Bring the puree and remaining water just to a boil in a large saucepan or teapot. Remove from heat and add the tea bags. Let steep for 7 minutes.

3. Remove the tea bags and refrigerate the tea until well chilled. Stir before serving over ice.

Exchanges: free; 10 calories, 0 calories from fat, 0 g total fat, 0 g saturated fat, 0 mg cholesterol, 0 mg sodium, 3 g total carbohydrate, 0 g dietary fiber, 2 g sugars, 0 g protein.

FRESH FACT

Blueberries top the list of fruits for total antioxidant power—and free radical-fighting ability. Other berries, including cranberries and raspberries, pack a punch, too. And, of course, all fruits provide beneficial nutrients.

FOOD FLAIR

Try raspberries or a mixture of berries in this recipe. Serve with a twist of lemon on the glass rim.

POMEGRANATE MARTINI

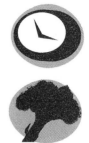

Serves 1/serving size: 1 martini

*This flavorful alcoholic drink is not a martini in the truest sense . . .
but when served in a martini glass, it sure looks like one.*

- 1/2 cup pomegranate juice, chilled
- 1 oz Grey Goose Le Citron vodka or other 80 proof lemon-flavored vodka, chilled (2 Tbsp)
- 1 oz sparkling water, chilled (2 Tbsp)
- 4 large ice cubes

DIRECTIONS

Add all ingredients to a shaker and shake, then strain into a chilled martini glass.

Exchanges: 1/2 carbohydrate plus 70 calories from alcohol; 140 calories, 0 calories from fat, 0 g total fat, 0 g saturated fat, 0 mg cholesterol, 15 mg sodium, 18 g total carbohydrate, 0 g dietary fiber, 17 g sugars, 1 g protein.

FAST FIX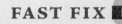

No shaker container . . . no problem!
Simply stir and enjoy.

FRESH FACT

Pomegranate juice contains a wealth of antioxidants. Research shows that it may improve blood flow to the heart and help lower blood pressure, too.

GAZPACHO COCKTAIL

Serves 4/serving size: 3/4 cup

This cocktail is made with tomato juice—a beverage loaded with lycopene. That's a carotenoid that makes tomatoes red. It may be beneficial for heart health and cancer prevention, too. Interestingly, processed tomato products, such as 100% tomato juice, have more lycopene than fresh tomatoes. So toast your health with this zippy, spicy nonalcoholic cocktail.

- 2 1/2 cups tomato juice (divided use)
- 1 1/2-inch piece English (hothouse) cucumber, roughly sliced
- 1/4 cup roughly sliced green onion
- 2 Tbsp lemon juice
- 2 tsp Worcestershire sauce
- 2 tsp aged red wine or balsamic vinegar
- 2 tsp prepared horseradish
- 1 large garlic clove
- 1/4 tsp hot pepper sauce, or to taste
- 4 Italian parsley sprigs

DIRECTIONS

1. Puree 1 cup tomato juice, cucumber, green onion, lemon juice, Worcestershire sauce, vinegar, horseradish, and garlic in a blender on low speed for 30 seconds, then high speed for 30 seconds or until smooth.

2. Pour into a pitcher. Stir in the remaining cups tomato juice and hot pepper sauce to taste. Refrigerate at least 1 hour to marry flavors. Serve chilled, with a parsley sprig in each glass.

Exchanges: 2 vegetable; 40 calories, 0 calories from fat, 0 g total fat, 0 g saturated fat, 0 mg cholesterol, 470 mg sodium, 9 g total carbohydrate, 2 g dietary fiber, 6 g sugars, 2 g protein.

FRESH FACT

Though full of nutrients, tomato juice is high in sodium. To help cut the sodium without negatively impacting flavor, mix 1 1/4 cups (10 oz) regular tomato juice with 1 1/4 cups (10 oz) low-sodium tomato juice.

FOOD FLAIR

Add leaves from an additional 4 (or more) parsley sprigs while pureeing for added fresh flavor. Serve in white wine glasses for extra elegance.

CITRUS WHITE SANGRIA

Serves 5/serving size: 3/4 cup

Sangria is a Spanish-inspired beverage traditionally made with red wine. But a bountiful pairing of fruit with white wine makes this an especially easy, cool, and breezy refresher for a warm day. Serve it over ice and sip.

- 1 fresh apricot or small nectarine, seeded and thinly sliced with peel
- 1 large navel orange, half sliced with peel, half juiced
- 1/4 cup fresh or frozen raspberries
- 1 (750-ml) bottle organic sauvignon blanc, pinot grigio, or riesling wine (with no added sulfites)

DIRECTIONS

1. Add the fruit slices and raspberries to a pitcher. Pour the orange juice and wine over the fruit and chill.

2. Serve the sangria chilled over ice, adding some of the fruit to each glass.

Exchanges: 1/2 carbohydrate plus 100 calories from alcohol; 150 calories, 0 calories from fat, 0 g total fat, 0 g saturated fat, 0 mg cholesterol, 10 mg sodium, 9 g total carbohydrate, 1 g dietary fiber, 5 g sugars, 0 g protein

FRESH FACT

Apricots and nectarines are seasonal in spring and summer. If it's fall or winter, leave them out of the sangria. Or use 1/3 cup frozen organic sliced peaches instead.

FAST FIX

You can make this recipe several hours ahead of time—in fact, it'll taste even fruitier. Just keep it covered and chilled until you're ready to serve.

FOOD FLAIR

Add 1 cup seltzer water to the pitcher of sangria just before serving—it provides zero calories of fun fizz!

SWEET ENDINGS

BALSAMIC STRAWBERRIES

Serves 4/serving size: 3/4 cup

Here, vinegar works like magic. It makes the strawberries surprisingly sweeter—without any added sugar!

- 1 lb strawberries, stems removed and sliced vertically
- 1 Tbsp aged balsamic, fig balsamic, or raspberry vinegar

DIRECTIONS

In a medium bowl, gently stir the strawberries and vinegar together. Serve at room temperature.

Exchanges: 1/2 fruit; 40 calories, 0 calories from fat, 0 g total fat, 0 g saturated fat, 0 mg cholesterol, 0 mg sodium, 9 g total carbohydrate, 2 g dietary fiber, 6 g sugars, 1 g protein.

FOOD FLAIR

If you prefer vibrant red strawberries, use the raspberry vinegar. The balsamic vinegar will slightly darken the strawberries. And for tastiest results, refrigerate these strawberries at least 2 hours before serving to allow them to marinate. Then bring to room temperature before serving.

WHIPPED BANANA SHERBET

Serves 4/serving size: 1/2 cup

When enjoying a sweet frozen treat, make your sugar calories count. When sugar comes naturally in the form of fruit, you're getting deliciousness along with nutrition. So, gather these ingredients and whip . . . whip it good!

- 3 medium fully ripened bananas, peeled and strings removed
- 1 tsp fresh lemon juice
- 1 tsp pure vanilla extract
- 1/8 tsp pure almond extract
- 1/2 cup plain soy milk

DIRECTIONS

1. Slice the bananas and place in a plastic freezer bag. Toss with lemon juice, seal, and freeze for 1 hour or until frozen solid.

2. Puree the banana slices, extracts, and soy milk in a blender until very smooth. Add additional soy milk by tablespoonfuls only if necessary.

3. Pour 1/2 cup banana puree into 4 small chilled glass dessert bowls. Cover and freeze for 2 hours or until solid.

Exchanges: 1 1/2 carbohydrate; 100 calories, 8 calories from fat, 1 g total fat, 0 g saturated fat, 0 mg cholesterol, 10 mg sodium, 23 g total carbohydrate, 3 g dietary fiber, 12 g sugars, 2 g protein.

FRESH FACT

When the banana peels are full of tiny brown "freckles," it means the bananas are fully ripened. That's when they're best for use in recipes, like this sherbet. When bananas aren't quite ripe, you can speed the process by sealing them in a brown paper bag at room temperature. The gasses released by the skins help the fruit ripen. This paper bag tip works with avocados, too.

GRILLED FRESH MISSION FIGS

Serves 4/serving size: 3 fig halves

Fresh figs are harvested from May through October—the ideal time of the year for outdoor grilling. So, get figgy with it at your next cookout. Figs make a gorgeous, gourmet accent to any cookout (or cook-in when the weather is frightful). Serve these fabulous figs as a dessert or, if you like, as an appetizer or side. They're succulent served with vanilla or lemon yogurt. And they're out of this world when paired with blue cheese.

- 6 medium fresh Black Mission figs
- 1 tsp aged balsamic vinegar
- 1 tsp acacia or orange blossom honey
- 2 tsp thinly sliced fresh mint

DIRECTIONS

1. Lightly coat a grill or grill pan with natural cooking spray. Preheat the grill or grill pan over medium-high heat. Remove stems from the figs and slice in half vertically.

2. Brush the cut surface of the figs with vinegar. Grill, cut side down, for about 3 minutes or until charred. Drizzle with honey and top with mint.

Exchanges: 1/2 fruit; 40 calories, 0 calories from fat, 0 g total fat, 0 g saturated fat, 0 mg cholesterol, 0 mg sodium, 10 g total carbohydrate, 1 g dietary fiber, 8 g sugars, 0 g protein.

FRESH FACT

A serving of figs has the highest overall mineral content of all common fruits. Plus, each serving provides more dietary fiber than any other common fresh or dried fruit.

FOOD FLAIR

Serve these figs topped with 3 Tbsp crumbled blue cheese. It's a classic combination—and a truly memorable mouthful. Then finish with a pinch of minced fresh rosemary instead of mint.

NEW-FASHIONED OATMEAL COOKIES

Serves 18/serving size: 1 cookie

Is it possible to have great-tasting cookies made with good-for-you ingredients, like whole grain oats and unsweetened applesauce? Whip up a batch of these new-fashioned, thin and crispy favorites and find out.

- 1 cup old-fashioned oats
- 1/2 cup unbleached all-purpose flour
- 1 1/2 tsp double-acting baking powder

- 3/4 tsp sea salt
- 3/4 cup turbinado sugar
- 3 Tbsp light brown sugar
- 3 Tbsp unsalted butter, room temperature

- 3 Tbsp organic unsweetened plain or cinnamon applesauce
- 1 large egg
- 1 1/2 tsp pure vanilla extract

DIRECTIONS

1. Preheat the oven to 350°F. In a small bowl, combine the oats, flour, baking powder, and salt.

2. Using an electric mixer at medium speed, cream the sugars and butter in a medium bowl. Add the applesauce, egg, and vanilla and blend until smooth. Add the dry mixture and blend until just combined.

3. Drop batter by rounded tablespoonfuls onto parchment paper-lined baking sheets about 2 inches apart. Bake for 22 minutes or until browned. Remove from the oven and let cool completely on the baking sheets. The cookies will crisp as they cool.

Exchanges: 1 carbohydrate, 1/2 fat; 90 calories, 22 calories from fat, 3 g total fat, 1 g saturated fat, 15 mg cholesterol, 150 mg sodium, 17 g total carbohydrate, 1 g dietary fiber, 10 g sugars, 2 g protein.

FRESH FACT

Whole oats are whole grains that contain soluble (or viscous) fiber, which can help reduce blood cholesterol levels. And in large quantities, soluble fiber may improve blood glucose control.

FOOD FLAIR

Add a pinch of ground cinnamon to the dry mixture. Cinnamon, considered a sweet spice, will add a bit of sweetness to these cookies without additional sugar. In fact, if you add cinnamon, go ahead and use 1 Tbsp less turbinado sugar in this recipe.

FAST FIX

Make your own oatmeal cookie mix. Measure the oats, flour, baking powder, and salt into a clean jar or sealable plastic bag. Label and date it. Store the mix in the pantry up to a couple of months. Make a few jars or bags of mix so you can bake cookies in a flash whenever you like.

POWER-PACKED PEANUT BUTTER COOKIES

Serves 30/serving size: 1 cookie

At less than 100 calories each, these cookies are a perfectly peanutty treat. Slowly savor every crispy, chewy bite.

- 1 cup unbleached all-purpose flour
- 1/3 cup whole wheat flour
- 1/2 tsp double-acting baking powder
- 1/2 tsp sea salt
- 2/3 cups natural chunky peanut butter
- 1/4 cup unsalted butter, room temperature
- 1 1/2 tsp pure vanilla extract
- 1/2 cup turbinado sugar
- 1/3 cup light brown sugar
- 1 large egg
- 2 Tbsp water

DIRECTIONS

1. Preheat the oven to 350°F. In a small bowl, combine the flours, baking powder, and salt. Using an electric mixer, blend the peanut butter, butter, and vanilla in a large bowl.

2. Add the sugars and blend, then add half the flour mixture and blend again. Add the egg and water and blend, then add the remaining flour mixture and blend again.

3. Form the dough into one large mound with your hands, then gently roll the dough into 30 small balls, about 1 rounded tablespoon of dough each.

4. Arrange the dough balls on parchment paper-lined baking sheets about 2 inches apart. Using the back of a fork, flatten the dough balls in a crosshatch design. Bake the cookies 22 minutes or until crisp. Cool cookies on the baking sheets for 5 minutes. Transfer cookies to racks and cool completely.

Exchanges: 1/2 carbohydrate, 1 fat; 90 calories, 41 calories from fat, 5 g total fat, 1 g saturated fat, 10 mg cholesterol, 70 mg sodium, 10 g total carbohydrate, 1 g dietary fiber, 6 g sugars, 2 g protein.

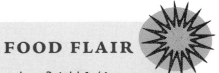

FOOD FLAIR

Want a cookie everyone will rave about? Add 1/4 cup turbinado sugar to a small bowl. Roll each cookie dough ball in the sugar, then continue with Step 4. If you like, roll part of them in sugar and leave the rest plain. The sugar-coated cookie has 10 more calories than its yummy cousin.

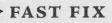

FAST FIX

You can make these cookies up to 3 days in advance and store them in an airtight container at room temperature—or freeze them up to 3 weeks.

CHILLY CHOCOLATE FONDUE

Serves 4/serving size: rounded 1/3 cup

This fondue is not really a fondue. But it acts like one here—just a chilled, velvety, chocolaty, and healthier version. Serve it with fresh strawberries, bananas, or other fresh fruit for dipping.

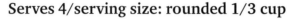

- 10 oz soft silken tofu, drained (1 rounded cup)
- 1/4 cup unsweetened natural cocoa powder
- 3 Tbsp chocolate soy milk
- 2 Tbsp acacia or other mild floral honey
- 1 tsp pure vanilla extract

DIRECTIONS

Puree all ingredients in a blender on low speed for 1 minute or until smooth. Pour into a serving bowl and chill at least 15 minutes before serving. Serve with fruit.

FOOD FLAIR

Instead of as a fondue, serve this dish as a pudding. It's gorgeous in small wine glasses.

Exchanges: 1 carbohydrate, 1/2 fat; 100 calories, 23 calories from fat, 3 g total fat, 0 g saturated fat, 0 mg cholesterol, 10 mg sodium, 15 g total carbohydrate, 1 g dietary fiber, 10 g sugars, 5 g protein.

FAST FIX

Make this fondue a day ahead of time. It actually tastes more delicious, since the flavors blend while chilling. Keep refrigerated until ready to serve.

JUST PEACHY BOWLS

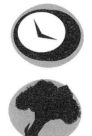

Serves 4/serving size: 1 bowl

These gorgeous "bowls" look so impressive, but they're really easy to prepare. They'll be simply divine when peaches are at their peak in spring or summer.

- 2 large fully ripened peaches
- 1 cup organic fat-free peach yogurt
- 2 Tbsp sliced almonds, pan-toasted
- 4 sprigs fresh mint

DIRECTIONS

1. Remove peach stems, slice peaches in half, and remove seeds. Place each peach half onto a small plate, cut side up. Top each half with 1/4 cup yogurt.

2. Sprinkle with almonds and top with mint sprigs.

Exchanges: 1 carbohydrate, 1/2 fat; 90 calories, 16 calories from fat, 2 g total fat, 0 g saturated fat, 0 mg cholesterol, 30 mg sodium, 16 g total carbohydrate, 2 g dietary fiber, 13 g sugars, 4 g protein.

FOOD FLAIR

Mix and match these refreshing bowls with various fresh fruit halves and yogurt flavors.

FAST FIX

Pan-toast 1/2 cup sliced almonds. Store the almonds in a sealed container in the refrigerator for weeks. They can be used for other recipes, too, like Fresh Tarragon Chicken Salad with Almonds on Marble Rye (see recipe, page 186).

FUDGY BROWNIES

Serves 25/serving size: 1 brownie

*These might be the best 100-calorie brownies you ever had!
You be the judge.*

- 1 1/2 cups turbinado sugar
- 1/3 cup canola oil
- 1/2 tsp sea salt
- 2 Tbsp water
- 1/4 cup unsweetened natural cocoa powder
- 3 oz high-quality unsweetened baking chocolate, chopped
- 4 large egg whites
- 2 tsp pure vanilla extract
- 1/3 cup unbleached all-purpose flour
- 1/3 cup whole wheat flour

DIRECTIONS

1. Preheat the oven to 375°F. Lightly coat a 9 × 13-inch nonstick baking pan with natural cooking spray.

2. In a large microwave-safe bowl, stir the sugar, oil, salt, and water together. Microwave on high power for 2 1/2 minutes or until the mixture rapidly bubbles, stirring once midway through the cooking time. (Be careful, as this mixture will be extremely hot.)

3. Stir in the cocoa and chocolate until the chocolate is melted. Vigorously stir in the egg whites one at a time and the vanilla. Stir in the flours until the batter is smooth.

4. Pour the batter into the pan and bake 18 minutes or until springy to the touch 1 inch from the edges. Cool completely in the pan. Cut into 25 pieces.

Exchanges: 1 carbohydrate, 1/2 fat; 100 calories, 43 calories from fat, 5 g total fat, 1 g saturated fat, 0 mg cholesterol, 55 mg sodium, 15 g total carbohydrate, 1 g dietary fiber, 12 g sugars, 2 g protein.

FRESH FACT

Chocolate can be good for the heart. But not all chocolate is created equal, health-wise. It's good news for some chocolate lovers, since the general rule is: the more bitter, the better. That means choose dark chocolate over milk chocolate. Luckily, these brownies fall into the delicious and nutritious dark category.

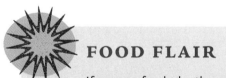

FOOD FLAIR

If you prefer, bake these chewy gems in an 8 × 8-inch nonstick baking pan for 20 minutes or until springy to the touch 1 inch from the edges. They'll be smaller squares, but much thicker.

MINI VANILLI CUPCAKES WITH CHERRIES ON TOP

Serves 36/serving size: 1 cupcake

Milli Vanilli, the musical duo, may not have been real. But these Mini Vanillis are 100% real. They're really good, too.

- 1 1/2 cups unbleached all-purpose flour
- 2 tsp double-acting baking powder
- 3/4 tsp sea salt
- 6 Tbsp unsalted butter, softened
- 1/3 cup canola oil
- 1 cup turbinado sugar
- 4 large egg whites
- 2 tsp pure vanilla extract (or 1 1/2 tsp pure vanilla extract and 1/2 tsp pure almond extract)
- 1/2 cup plain soy milk
- 18 Bing (sweet) cherries, pitted and halved

DIRECTIONS

1. Preheat the oven to 325°F. Line 3 (12-capacity) mini-muffin tins with mini-muffin/cupcake papers. In a small bowl, combine the flour, baking powder, and salt.

2. Using an electric mixer, blend the butter in a large bowl until smooth. Add the oil and blend until smooth. Add the sugar and beat for 1 minute.

3. Add the egg whites and vanilla and beat for 1 minute. Add half the dry ingredients, then half the soy milk. Beat until thoroughly combined, then repeat.

4. Spoon 1 heaping tablespoon batter into each cupcake liner, filling about 7/8 full. Gently place 1 cherry half on top of each, cut side down. Bake for 18 minutes or until a toothpick inserted in the cupcake comes out clean.

5. Cool cupcakes in the tins for 10 minutes, then remove from tins and cool completely on racks.

Exchanges: 1/2 carbohydrate, 1 fat; 80 calories, 36 calories from fat, 4 g total fat, 1 g saturated fat, 5 mg cholesterol, 85 mg sodium, 10 g total carbohydrate, 0 g dietary fiber, 6 g sugars, 1 g protein.

FRESH FACT

Halve cherries just like you halve avocados. Slice vertically all the way around while touching the seed with your knife. Twist and separate into halves, then remove the seed.

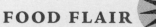

FOOD FLAIR

Bake these without the cherries, let cool, then frost as you wish for a kids' (or adults') party. They're the perfect size for pint-sized appetites or finger-food noshing.

RESOURCES

WHAT'S IN SEASON?

WINTER (December, January, February)

Fruits

Apple
Avocado/Hass avocado
Banana
Cherimoya
Date
Grape
Grapefruit
Guava
Kiwifruit
Kumquat

Lemon/Meyer lemon
Mango
Orange: blood, navel
Papaya
Pear: Anjou, Bartlett, Bosc,
  Comice, Seckel
Plantain
Pomelo
Quince
Starfruit
Tangerine/Mandarin orange

Vegetables

Artichoke	Mushroom/wild mushroom
Asparagus	Onion: Spanish (common
Broccoli	yellow), green (scallion)
Broccoli rabe	Parsley
Cabbage: bok choy, red/green/	Parsnip
white, Brussels sprouts, Napa	Pepper: chili, sweet bell
Carrot	Potato: russet, fingerling
Cauliflower	Potato: sweet
Celeriac/celery root	Radicchio
Celery	Radish: Daikon
Chard	Rutabaga
Chestnut	Shallot
Endive: Belgian (chicory), curly	Spinach
Fennel	Squash: winter
Garlic	Sunchoke
Greens: collard, dandelion, kale,	Taro
mustard, turnip	Tomatillo
Jicama	Turnip
Leek	Watercress
Lettuce	Yuca

SPRING (March, April, May)

Fruits

Apricot	Mango
Avocado/Hass avocado	Nectarine
Banana	Orange: navel
Berries: blueberries, strawberries	Papaya
Cherimoya	Peach
Grape	Pear: Anjou, Bosc
Grapefruit	Pineapple
Kiwifruit	Plantain
Kumquat	Rhubarb
Lemon	Tangerine

Vegetables

Artichoke
Asparagus
Beans, shell: fava
Beet
Broccoli
Cabbage: bok choy, red/green/
  white, Napa
Carrot
Cauliflower
Celeriac/celery root
Chard
Corn
Fennel
Endive: curly
Garlic
Ginger
Greens: collard, dandelion,
  kale, mustard, Swiss chard
Jicama
Leek
Lettuce

Mushrooms/morels
Nopales
Onion: red, green (scallion),
  Vidalia
Pea: garden, sugar-snap, snow
Pepper: chili, sweet bell
Potato: russet, new, fingerling,
  long whites
Radish
Ramp
Rutabaga
Shallot
Sorrel
Spinach
Squash: summer
  (including zucchini)
Sunchoke
Taro
Tomatillo
Watercress
Yuca

SUMMER (June, July, August)

Fruits

Apricot
Avocado
Banana
Berries: blackberries,
  boysenberries, loganberries,
  marionberries, blueberries,
  raspberries, strawberries
Cherry
Currant

Fig: Black Mission, Brown
  Turkey, Calimyrna, Kadota
Grape
Guava
Lemon
Lime: Key
Loquat
Lychee
Mango

Melon: cantaloupe, honeydew,
  watermelon
Nectarine
Orange: Valencia
Papaya

Peach
Pear: Asian
Pineapple
Plantain
Plum

Vegetables

Basil
Beans, shell: cranberry, lima
Beet
Cabbage: bok choy, red/green/
  white, Napa
Corn
Cucumber
Edamame
Eggplant
Garlic
Ginger
Green beans
Greens: arugula, mustard,
  Swiss chard
Jicama
Lettuce
Mushrooms

Okra
Onion: red, pearl, green
  (scallion), Vidalia, Walla Walla
Pea: garden, sugar-snap, snow
Pepper: chili, sweet bell
Potato: russet, new, Yukon gold
Ramp
Shallot
Spinach
Squash: summer
  (including zucchini)
Taro
Tomatillo
Tomato
Water chestnut
Watercress
Yuca

FALL (September, October, November)

Fruits

Apple
Avocado
Banana
Berries: cranberries, raspberries
Fig: Black Mission, Brown
  Turkey, Kadota
Grape

Kiwi
Mango
Melon: cantaloupe
Orange: Valencia, navel
Papaya
Pear: Anjou, Asian, Bartlett,
  Bosc, Comice, Seckel

Persimmon
Plantain
Plum

Pomegranate
Quince
Starfruit

Vegetables

Artichoke
Basil
Beet
Broccoli
Cabbage: bok choy, red/green/
  white, Savoy, Brussels
  sprouts, Napa
Carrot
Celeriac/celery root
Celery
Chard
Chestnut
Cucumber
Dill
Eggplant
Garlic
Green beans
Greens: arugula, turnip,
  Swiss chard
Jicama
Leek
Lettuce
Mushrooms
Okra

Onion: pearl, green (scallion),
  Spanish (common yellow)
Parsley
Parsnip
Pepper: chili, sweet bell
Potato: russet, blue/purple,
  fingerlings, Russian banana,
  sweet, Yukon gold
Pumpkin
Radish: Daikon
Rutabaga
Shallot
Spinach
Squash: winter
Sunchoke
Taro
Tomatillo
Tomato
Turnip
Water chestnut
Watercress
Yam
Yuca

DIABETES INFORMATION

American Diabetes Association
www.diabetes.org
800-DIABETES (800-342-2383)

The American Dietetic Association
www.eatright.org
312-899-0040

American Association of Diabetes Educators
www.aadenet.org
800-338-3633

American Academy of Family Physicians
www.familydoctor.org
800-274-2237

American Heart Association
www.americanheart.org
800-AHA-USA1 (800-242-8721)

**Centers for Disease Control and Prevention/
National Center for Chronic Disease Prevention and
Health Promotion**
www.cdc.gov/diabetes
800-CDC-INFO (800-232-4636)

**Diabetes Care and Education Dietetic Practice Group
(of The American Dietetic Association)**
www.dce.org

Federación Española de Asociaciones de Educadores
en Diabetes (FEAED)
(The Spanish Federation of Association of Educators in Diabetes)
www.feaed.org

International Diabetes Federation
www.idf.org

National Diabetes Education Program
www.ndep.nih.gov
800-438-5383

National Heart, Lung, and Blood Institute
www.nhlbi.nih.gov
301-592-8573

National Institute of Diabetes and Digestive and Kidney
Diseases/National Diabetes Information Clearinghouse
www.niddk.nih.gov
www.diabetes.niddk.nih.gov
800-860-8747

WebMD®/Diabetes Health Center (online only)
http://diabetes.webmd.com

World Health Organization/Diabetes Unit
www.who.int/diabetes/en

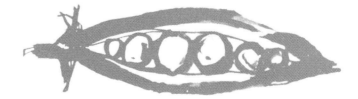

NATURAL FOODS: ONLINE LINKS

GreenPeople
www.greenpeople.org

**HappyCow's Vegetarian Guide to Restaurants &
Health Food Stores**
www.happycow.net/north_america/usa/

Local Harvest
www.localharvest.org

National Green Pages
www.coopamerica.org/pubs/greenpages

Natural Food Network
www.naturalfoodnet.com

Organic Consumers Association
www.organicconsumers.org/btc/BuyingGuide.cfm

Sustainable Table/Eat Well Guide
www.eatwellguide.org

The New Farm/Farm Locator
www.newfarm.org/farmlocator

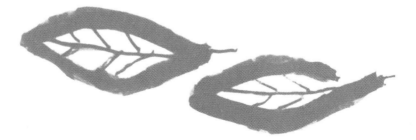

WEBSITES FOR FOOD INFORMATION

Almonds
Almond Board of California
www.almondsarein.com

Apples
U.S. Apple Association
www.usapple.org

Asparagus
California Asparagus Commission
www.calasparagus.com

Avocados
California Avocado Commission
www.avocado.org
Hass Avocado Board
www.avocadocentral.com

Bananas
International Banana Association
www.eatmorebananas.com

Beans
American Dry Bean Board
www.americanbean.org

Beef
National Cattlemen's Beef Association
www.beef.org

Beer
National Beer Wholesalers of America
www.nbwa.org/Nbwa/home_public.htm

Blueberries
North American Blueberry Council
  www.blueberry.org

Cheese (see Dairy)

Cherries
California Cherry Advisory Board
  www.calcherry.com
Cherry Marketing Institute
  www.choosecherries.com

Chicken/Poultry
National Chicken Council and U.S. Poultry & Egg Association
  www.eatchicken.com

Chocolate
Chocolate Manufacturers Association
  www.chocolateusa.org

Cranberries
Cranberry Marketing Committee
  www.uscranberries.com

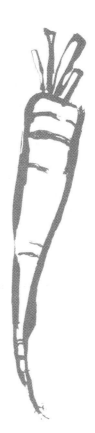

Dairy
National Dairy Council
  www.nationaldairycouncil.org
3-A-Day™ of Dairy
  www.3aday.org

Eggs
American Egg Board
  www.aeb.org
Egg Nutrition Center
www.enc-online.org

Figs
California Fig Advisory Board
  www.californiafigs.com

Fish/Seafood
National Fisheries Institute, Inc.
  www.aboutseafood.com

Flaxseed
Flax Council of Canada
  www.flaxcouncil.ca

Fruit/Tree Fruit (peaches, plums, nectarines)
California Tree Fruit Agreement
  www.eatcaliforniafruit.com

Grains/Wheat
Kansas Wheat Commission
  www.kswheat.com
Wheat Foods Council
  www.wheatfoods.org

Grapes
California Table Grape Commission
  www.tablegrape.com

Greens
Leafy Greens Council
  www.leafy-greens.org

Hazelnuts
The Hazelnut Council
  www.hazelnutcouncil.org

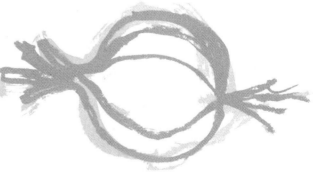

Honey
National Honey Board
  www.honey.com

Lamb
American Lamb Board
  www.americanlamb.com

Lentils
USA Dry Peas, Lentils, & Chickpeas
  www.pea-lentil.com

Maple Syrup
Maine Maple Producers Association
  www.mainemapleproducers.com

Meat
American Meat Institute
  www.meatami.org

Milk (see Dairy)

Nuts
International Tree Nut Council
  www.nuthealth.org

Oil, Canola
Canola Council of Canada
  www.canola-council.org

Oil, Olive
California Olive Oil Council
  www.cooc.com
Trade Commission of Spain
  www.oliveoilfromspain.com

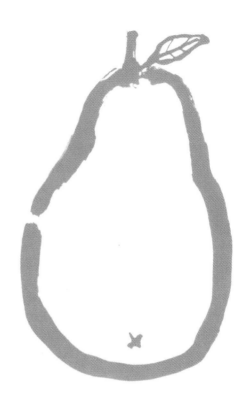

Onions
National Onion Association
  www.onions-usa.org
The Vidalia Onion Committee
  www.vidaliaonion.org

Pasta
National Pasta Association
  www.ilovepasta.org

Peanuts
The Peanut Institute
  www.peanut-institute.org

Peanut Butter
Peanut Advisory Board
  www.peanutbutterlovers.com

Pears
Pear Bureau Northwest
  www.usapears.com

Pecans
National Pecan Shellers Association
  www.ilovepecans.org

Pistachios
California Pistachio Commission
  www.pistachios.org

Plums, Dried
California Dried Plum Board
  www.californiadriedplums.org

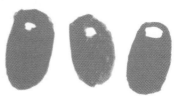

Pork
National Pork Board
  www.theotherwhitemeat.com

Potatoes
United States Potato Board
  www.healthypotato.com

Produce
Produce for Better Health Foundation
  www.5aday.com

Raspberries
Washington Red Raspberry Commission
  www.red-raspberry.org

Rice
USA Rice Federation
  www.riceinfo.com

Soy
United Soybean Board
  www.talksoy.com

Spirits
Distilled Spirits Council of the United States
  www.discus.org

Strawberries
California Strawberry Commission
  www.calstrawberry.com

Sugar
The Sugar Association
  www.sugar.org

Sweet Potatoes
The United States Sweet Potato Council, Inc.
  www.sweetpotatousa.org

Tea
Tea Council of the U.S.A.
  www.teausa.org

Tomatoes
California Tomato Commission
  www.tomato.org
Florida Tomato Committee
  www.floridatomatoes.org
Processed Tomato Foundation
  www.tomatonet.org

Turkey
National Turkey Federation
  www.eatturkey.com

Vinegar
The Vinegar Institute
  www.versatilevinegar.org

Walnuts
Walnut Marketing Board
  www.walnut.org

Wine
American Wine Society
  www.americanwinesociety.org

ADDITIONAL INFORMATION ABOUT FOOD

The American Institute of Wine & Food
www.aiwf.org

Calorie Control Council
www.caloriecontrol.org

Environmental Defense
www.environmentaldefense.org

Environmental Working Group
www.ewg.org

Food Marketing Institute
www.fmi.org

Green Restaurant Association
www.dinegreen.com

**Grocery Manufacturers Association/
Food Processors Association**
www.gmabrands.com

HarvestEating.com
www.harvesteating.com

Healthy Children Healthy Futures
www.healthychildrenhealthyfutures.org

International Food Information Council
www.ific.org
www.kidnetic.com

The James Beard Foundation
www.jamesbeard.org

National Fiber Council
www.nationalfibercouncil.org

National Restaurant Association/Healthy Dining Finder
www.healthydiningfinder.com

National Sustainable Agriculture Information Service
www.attra.org

Natural Products Association
www.naturalproductsassoc.org

Natural Products Expo East/Organic Products Expo
www.expoeast.com

Natural Products Expo West
www.expowest.com

North American Farmers' Direct Marketing Association
www.nafdma.com

Organic Trade Association
www.ota.com

Partnership for Food Safety Education/Fight Bac!
www.fightbac.org

Slow Food
www.slowfood.com

Turkey Talk-Line
www.butterball.com
800-BUTTERBALL or 800-288-8372

**USDA/Agricultural Marketing Service/
Farmer Direct Marketing**
www.ams.usda.gov/directmarketing

**USDA/National Agricultural Library/
Food and Nutrition Information Center**
http://fnic.nal.usda.gov

USDA/Meat and Poultry Hotline
www.fsis.usda.gov/Food_Safety_Education/USDA_Meat_&_
Poultry_Hotline
888-MPHotline or 888-674-6854

USDA/MyPyramid.gov
www.mypyramid.gov

The Vegetarian Resource Group
www.vrg.org

COOKING AND HEALTHY EATING/LIFESTYLE PUBLICATIONS AND ONLINE RESOURCES

American Diabetes Association (includes online store)
www.diabetes.org
www.diabetes.org/shop-for-books-and-gifts.jsp

Diabetes Forecast Magazine

www.diabetes.org/diabetes-forecast.jsp

Active Interest Media
www.aimmedia.com
www.betternutrition.com
www.vegetariantimes.com

Allrecipes.com
www.allrecipes.com

Amazon.com
www.amazon.com

America's Test Kitchen
www.americastestkitchen.com
www.cookscountry.com
www.cooksillustrated.com

American Express Publishing Corporation
www.amexpub.com
www.foodandwine.com
www.travelandleisure.com/family

August Home Publishing Company
www.augusthome.com
www.cuisineathome.com

Barnes & Noble
www.bn.com

Bauer Publishing
www.bauerpublishing.com
www.myfirstforwomen.com

Chocolatier Magazine
www.chocolatiermagazine.com

CondéNet
www.condenet.com
www.bonappetit.com
www.epicurious.com
www.glamour.com
www.gourmet.com
www.houseandgarden.com
www.janemag.com
www.nutritiondata.com
www.self.com

Discovery Health
http://health.discovery.com

Food Network
www.foodnetwork.com

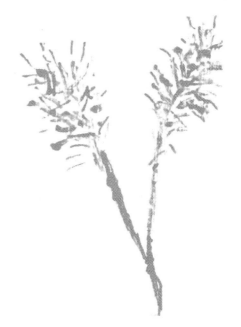

Great Valley Publishing Co., Inc.
www.gvpub.com
www.todaysdietandnutrition.com

Hachette Filipacchi Media U.S., Inc.
www.hfmus.com
www.womansday.com

Hearst Magazines
www.hearst.com/magazines
www.countryliving.com
www.goodhousekeeping.com
www.marieclaire.com
www.oprah.com/omagazine
www.quickandsimple.com
www.redbookmag.com
www.seventeen.com

LifeMed Media
www.dlife.com

Meredith Corporation
www.meredith.com
www.bhg.com
www.familycircle.com
www.fitnessmagazine.com
www.lhj.com
www.midwestliving.com
www.more.com
www.parents.com

ParadeNet Inc.
www.parade.com

Recipe4Living
www.recipe4living.com

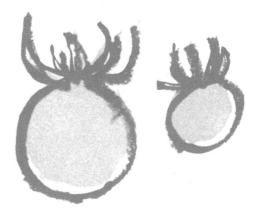

Rodale Magazines International
www.rodale.com
www.menshealth.com
www.organicgardening.com
www.prevention.com
www.womenshealthmag.com

The Taunton Press
www.taunton.com
www.finecooking.com
www.finegardening.com

Time Inc.
www.pathfinder.com
www.coastalliving.com
www.cookinglight.com
www.health.com
www.myrecipes.com
www.realsimple.com
www.southernliving.com
www.sunset.com

Weider Publications
www.fitnessonline.com
www.mensfitness.com
www.naturalhealthmag.com
www.shape.com

Weight Watchers International
www.weightwatchers.com

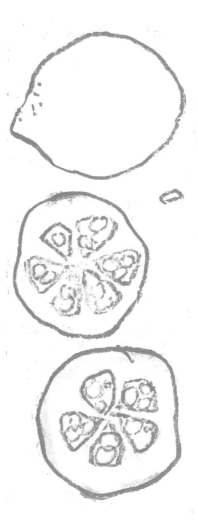

MEASUREMENT EQUIVALENCIES

Weights and Measures Equivalencies

3 teaspoons (tsp)	=	1 tablespoon (Tbsp) (1/2 fl oz)
1/2 Tbsp	=	1 1/2 tsp
2 Tbsp	=	1/8 cup (1 fl oz)
4 Tbsp	=	1/4 cup (2 fl oz)
5 1/3 Tbsp	=	1/3 cup; 5 Tbsp + 1 tsp
8 Tbsp	=	1/2 cup (4 fl oz)
10 2/3 Tbsp	=	2/3 cup; 10 Tbsp + 2 tsp
12 Tbsp	=	3/4 cup (6 fl oz)
16 Tbsp	=	1 cup (8 fl oz)
2 cups	=	1 pint (16 fl oz)
2 pints	=	1 quart; 4 cups (32 fl oz)
4 quarts	=	1 gallon; 8 pints; 16 cups (128 fl oz)

Metric Weights and Measures Equivalencies

1 gram (g)	=	1/28 oz (0.035 oz)
1/2 oz	=	15 g
1 oz	=	30 g
2 oz	=	60 g
4 oz	=	110 g
6 oz	=	170 g
8 oz	=	225 g
12 oz	=	340 g
16 oz (1 lb)	=	450 g
2.2 lbs	=	1 kilogram (kg)
35 fl oz	=	1 liter (l)

METRIC CONVERSION CHART

Measurement	Convert to	Multiply by
ounces (oz)	grams (g)	28.35
pounds (lb)	kilograms (kg)	0.45
teaspoons (tsp)	milliliters (ml)	5
tablespoons (Tbsp)	milliliters (ml)	15
fluid ounces (fl oz)	milliliters (ml)	30
cups	liters (l)	0.24
pints (pt)	liters (l)	0.47
quarts (qt)	liters (l)	0.95

INDEX

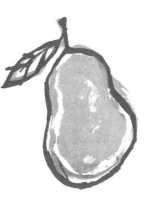

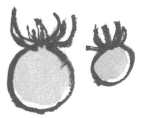

QUICK-TO-FIX RECIPES

VEGETARIAN RECIPES

Other Titles Available from the American Diabetes Association

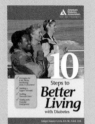

10 Steps to Better Living with Diabetes
by Ginger Kanzer-Lewis, RN, BC, EdM, CDE
Don't let diabetes take control of your life. Instead, take control of your diabetes! Learn the answers to all of your questions about self-care, including the questions you didn't even know to ask. Start living a better life with diabetes—let Ginger Kanzer-Lewis show you how.
Order no. 4882-01; Price $16.95

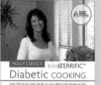

The Diabetes Dictionary
by American Diabetes Association
To stay healthy, you need to understand the constantly growing vocabulary of diabetes research and treatment. This gives you the straightforward definitions of diabetes terms and concepts you need. With more than 500 entries, this affordable, pocket-size book is an indispensable resource for every person with diabetes.
Order no. 5020-01; Price $5.95

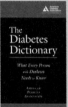

Holly Clegg's Trim & Terrific™ Diabetic Cooking
by Holly Clegg
Cookbook author Holly Clegg has teamed up with the American Diabetes Association to create a Trim & Terrific™ cookbook perfect for people with diabetes. With over 250 recipes, this collection is packed with meals that are quick, easy, and delicious. Forget the hassles of meal planning and rediscover the joys of great food!
Order no. 4883-01; Price $18.95

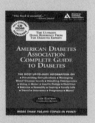

American Diabetes Association Complete Guide to Diabetes, 4th Edition
by American Diabetes Association
Have all the information on diabetes that you need close at hand. The world's largest collection of diabetes self-care tips, techniques, and tricks for solving diabetes-related problems is back in its fourth edition, and it's bigger and better than ever before.
Order no. 4809-04; Price $29.95

To order these and other great American Diabetes Association titles, call 1-800-232-6733 or visit http://store.diabetes.org.
American Diabetes Association titles are also available in bookstores nationwide.

About the American Diabetes Association

The American Diabetes Association is the nation's leading voluntary health organization supporting diabetes research, information, and advocacy. Its mission is to prevent and cure diabetes and to improve the lives of all people affected by diabetes. The American Diabetes Association is the leading publisher of comprehensive diabetes information. Its huge library of practical and authoritative books for people with diabetes covers every aspect of self-care—cooking and nutrition, fitness, weight control, medications, complications, emotional issues, and general self-care.

To order American Diabetes Association books: Call 1-800-232-6733 or log on to *http://store.diabetes.org*

To join the American Diabetes Association: Call 1-800-806-7801 or log on to *www.diabetes.org/membership*

For more information about diabetes or ADA programs and services: Call 1-800-342-2383. E-mail: AskADA@diabetes.org or log on to *www.diabetes.org*

To locate an ADA/NCQA Recognized Provider of quality diabetes care in your area: *www.ncqa. org/dprp*

To find an ADA Recognized Education Program in your area: Call 1-800-342-2383. *www.diabetes.org/for-health-professionals-and-scientists/recognition/edrecognition.jsp*

To join the fight to increase funding for diabetes research, end discrimination, and improve insurance coverage: Call 1-800-342-2383. *www.diabetes.org/advocacy-and-legalresources/advocacy.jsp*

To find out how you can get involved with the programs in your community: Call 1-800-342-2383. See below for program Web addresses.

- *American Diabetes Month:* educational activities aimed at those diagnosed with diabetes—month of November. *www.diabetes.org/communityprograms-and-localevents/americandiabetesmonth.jsp*
- *American Diabetes Alert:* annual public awareness campaign to find the undiagnosed—held the fourth Tuesday in March. *www.diabetes.org/communityprograms-and-localevents/americandiabetesalert.jsp*
- *American Diabetes Association Latino Initiative:* diabetes awareness program targeted to the Latino community. *www.diabetes.org/communityprograms-and-localevents/latinos.jsp*
- *African American Program:* diabetes awareness program targeted to the African American community. *www.diabetes.org/communityprograms-and-localevents/africanamericans.jsp*
- *Awakening the Spirit: Pathways to Diabetes Prevention & Control:* diabetes awareness program targeted to the Native American community. *www.diabetes.org/communityprograms-and-localevents/nativeamericans.jsp*

To find out about an important research project regarding type 2 diabetes: *www.diabetes.org/diabetes-research/research-home.jsp*

To obtain information on making a planned gift or charitable bequest: Call 1-888-700-7029. *www.wpg.cc/stl/CDA/homepage/1,1006,509,00.html*

To make a donation or memorial contribution: Call 1-800-342-2383. *www.diabetes.org/support-the-cause/make-a-donation.jsp*